AF147564

Pain, Drugs, and Ethics

Kevin L. Zacharoff · Phyllis Migdal

Pain, Drugs, and Ethics

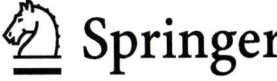 Springer

Kevin L. Zacharoff
Department of Family, Population, and
Preventive Medicine
Renaissance School of Medicine at Stony
Brook University
Stony Brook, NY, USA

Phyllis Migdal
Department of Family, Population, and
Preventive Medicine
Renaissance School of Medicine at Stony
Brook University
Stony Brook, NY, USA

ISBN 978-3-031-63017-0   ISBN 978-3-031-63018-7   (eBook)
https://doi.org/10.1007/978-3-031-63018-7

© The Editor(s) (if applicable) and The Author(s), under exclusive license to Springer Nature Switzerland AG 2024

This work is subject to copyright. All rights are solely and exclusively licensed by the Publisher, whether the whole or part of the material is concerned, specifically the rights of translation, reprinting, reuse of illustrations, recitation, broadcasting, reproduction on microfilms or in any other physical way, and transmission or information storage and retrieval, electronic adaptation, computer software, or by similar or dissimilar methodology now known or hereafter developed.

The use of general descriptive names, registered names, trademarks, service marks, etc. in this publication does not imply, even in the absence of a specific statement, that such names are exempt from the relevant protective laws and regulations and therefore free for general use.

The publisher, the authors and the editors are safe to assume that the advice and information in this book are believed to be true and accurate at the date of publication. Neither the publisher nor the authors or the editors give a warranty, expressed or implied, with respect to the material contained herein or for any errors or omissions that may have been made. The publisher remains neutral with regard to jurisdictional claims in published maps and institutional affiliations.

This Springer imprint is published by the registered company Springer Nature Switzerland AG
The registered company address is: Gewerbestrasse 11, 6330 Cham, Switzerland

If disposing of this product, please recycle the paper.

This book is dedicated to our students, who give us hope for a better and more compassionate future.

Preface

Pain, Drugs, and Ethics is the culmination of years of personal observation and involvement with the implementation of numerous clinical and regulatory approaches and measures which have significantly impacted how pain is assessed and managed. During this time, I have observed wide and pendulous shifts in public opinion, clinical practice recommendations, and guideline deployment. This has been particularly evident with respect to the use of opioid analgesics in the management of acute and chronic pain. In some instances, the result of these shifts has been to make what were once considered clinically acceptable or desirable treatment options offered to people with pain, to then be considered undesirable, inappropriate, and in some cases worthy of regulatory scrutiny. Additionally, I have witnessed other factors which have the potential to significantly affect how people with pain are treated remain unchanged. These include bias, stigma, social determinants of health, and the emergence and persistence of the overdose epidemic plaguing the United States today. A large part of the impetus for authoring this book was that the tumultuous world of pain and its management seems to have negatively impacted the ability to maintain focus on the ethical mandate to compassionately treat those in pain and alleviate their suffering.

I have often been frustrated by the fact that despite pain being one of the single most common reasons that people seek medical attention, healthcare professional education about its assessment and treatment has been and continues to be sparse, fragmented, or absent across healthcare professional training programs. In fact, it has not been uncommon for me to witness respected pain and/or substance use experts in both clinical and public policymaking settings express that when it comes to pain and its management, "education does not make a difference." Certainly, there has been substantial debate related to this—but if we *are* willing to agree that education *can* be effective in improving the safety and quality of pain management, the question then remains as to how we can best provide education to the degree and breadth of dissemination possible to effectively achieve these goals.

Key intentions of this book are to inspire thought, instill a desire to acquire more knowledge, and also consider these often highly charged subjects rationally. We need to turn these topics into educational opportunities to help us better identify and understand the relationship between pain, drugs, and ethics. By using ethics as our guide, I believe that we can reliably approach those in pain as individuals, worthy of objective, equitable, and compassionate care in a way that can potentially achieve many things but really just help us to do one thing—care for patients suffering from pain in the safest and most effective way possible.

Along our organic and collaborative journey together, Dr. Migdal and I have learned many things, including the importance of educating students and clinicians about the dynamic and intimate relationship between pain, suffering, substance use, bias, stigma, social determinants of health, and healthcare disparities. My hope is that this book will help the reader gain a greater degree of stability and sense of confidence in pain assessment and its treatment, to better understand the role of opioid analgesic therapy in caring for people with pain when appropriate, and to better navigate challenges associated with the continuing epidemic of overdose fatalities and substance use.

Our goal is to help facilitate the delivery of compassionate, empathetic, and equitable care to patients in need. This includes not only people with pain, but also those with addiction or substance use disorders. What is most important to me personally is the possibility that this book can help you come to the same realization that I had: that the most valuable, consistent, and reproducible strategies we have to achieve those goals is also one of the oldest—letting ethics be our guide. Remember, there is no ethical pendulum.

Stony Brook, NY, USA   Kevin L. Zacharoff

Preface

My involvement in *Pain, Drugs, and Ethics* began several years ago when Dr. Zacharoff asked me to collaborate with him to educate medical students on this subject. These lectures involved the intersection of pain, bias, stigma, and the social determinants of health. This curriculum has evolved across all 4 years of medical school providing a longitudinal learning experience for the medical students.

Understanding how to treat patients with pain and provide effective care requires that we consider the effects of social and structural forces on individuals. Ethics underlies each of these issues as we strive to provide an educational groundwork for students and other healthcare professionals to not only gain knowledge about the treatment of pain, but to do so with understanding and compassion.

Patients experiencing pain may be considered "difficult" by health professionals, and this is not necessarily because of the discomfort, suffering, or daily impact of acute or chronic pain on the individual. Some physicians state that they get frustrated by these patients and do not feel comfortable seeing them, especially if they require opioid medication or have a history of substance use disorder. This frustration reflects a sad reality: physicians do lack the appropriate education and training to manage persons with pain in their day-to-day practices. Yet, if the goal of medicine is to achieve health and prevent or stabilize disease, isn't this the group of patients that most needs well-informed and compassionate care, built through a strong and trusting physician–patient relationship?

Education grounds the discussion of pain, drugs, and ethics. Raising awareness of the impact of outside influences, like media and regulatory agencies on the treatment of pain, and deepening understanding of the multilevel factors that influence these patients is key. This has been the goal of our educational practices and is the purpose of this book. It is my hope that understanding the multifaceted influences on the care of people with pain, including personal biases that we all harbor but may not be aware of, stigma that may profoundly affect the individual in pain and their access to care, the influence of the social determinants of health, and the institutional and structural factors that influence treatment, will improve the care of these patients.

In 1926, during an address at the Harvard School of Medicine, Dr. Frances Peabody stated, "One of the essential qualities of the clinician is interest in humanity, for the secret of care of the patient is in caring for the patient" [1]. To overcome the obstacles of caring for the patient in pain, we must seek out additional education, expand our knowledge, and increase awareness about this complex issue. Connecting with patients as expressed by Dr. Peabody will allow us to build trust and to provide more compassionate care, ultimately leading to a more effective and equitable treatment of pain. The sentiment embodies the importance of remaining open to the value of education and awareness about the treatment of pain. If we are more able to incorporate this ideal in our practice as we gain awareness about the complexities of this issue, then we can realize our goals of improving pain treatment and decreasing disparities in our care of this vulnerable group of patients.

Stony Brook, NY, USA   Phyllis Migdal

Reference

1. Peabody FW. The care of the patient. JAMA. 1927;88(12):877–82.

Contents

About the Authors

Kevin L. Zacharoff Dr. Kevin L. Zacharoff is a Board-Certified Anesthesiologist with over 25 years of clinical experience in Anesthesiology, Pediatric Anesthesiology, and Pain Medicine. He is an active Faculty Member and Clinical Assistant Professor at the Renaissance School of Medicine at Stony Brook University in the Department of Family, Population and Preventive Medicine, serves as the Course Director for Pain and Addiction at the medical school, and is a Distinguished Visiting Scholar in the Center for Medical Humanities, Compassionate Care, and Bioethics at Stony Brook. He has been particularly devoted to the examination of ethical issues involving pain management and substance use, providing education on these topics, and involved in research in these areas for more than 20 years. He has authored several texts including *The PainEUD.Org Manual: A Pocket Guide to Pain Management, Your Guide to Pain Management, Cross-Cultural Pain Management: Effective Treatment of Pain in the Hispanic Population,* and *Managing Chronic Pain with Opioids in Primary Care*; written several peer-reviewed journal articles; and most recently (2023) authored a chapter in the textbook *Sex and Gender Effects in Pharmacology* titled "Sex Differences in Pain and Its Treatment." Dr. Zacharoff has served as a co-investigator for several NIH-grant-funded research projects in the areas of pain, substance use, and the education of patients and clinicians on these topics. In addition to lecturing nationally on these subjects, Dr. Zacharoff has been involved in public policy, recently completing a 4-year term as a member of the Anesthetic and Analgesic Drug Products Advisory Committee to the United States Food and Drug Administration and currently serving as a consultant to this Committee. He has served as the Editor-in-Chief of *The PAINWeek Journal* and currently serves on the editorial review board of several peer-reviewed journals including *The Journal of Pain, Pain Medicine, The British Medical Journal, Pharmacoepidemiology and Drug Safety,* and *The Journal of Addictive Diseases.*

Phyllis Migdal Phyllis Migdal, MD, MA, is a faculty member in the Center for Medical Humanities, Compassionate Care, and Bioethics at the Renaissance School of Medicine at Stony Brook (SOM). As a Clinical Assistant Professor, she teaches in the master's program and in the medical school in the *Medicine in Contemporary Society* (MCS) course. Dr. Migdal is a frequent guest lecturer with focus on clinical ethics and the influence of social determinants of health, stigma, and bias on the persistence of health disparity. She also participates as a facilitator for Reflection

Rounds with pediatric residents and with medical students during their clerkship years. With a strong interest in medical ethics, she is a member of the Institutional Ethics Committee, including being active in hospital ethics consultation and serving on the educational subcommittee. Her interests further include fostering compassionate care in physician training, the clinical practice of bioethical decision-making, and increasing the awareness of the impact of stigma and bias on the care of patients.

Prior to joining the faculty in 2018, Dr. Migdal practiced clinical endocrinology in the Stony Brook community after completing medical school, residency, and fellowship in Endocrinology and Metabolism in 1997 at Stony Brook University Hospital. While in private practice, she was a preceptor for medical students and residents and led educational workshops for diabetics. She graduated summa cum laude from New York University in 1982 and completed her master's degree in Medical Humanities, Compassionate Care and Bioethics at Stony Brook University in 2018.

The Conundrum of Pain

1

Background

Over the course of my clinical and educational career and even in my pre-clinical education, I have found people's impressions about pain to be quite interesting, quite varied, and quite passionate—with an extra helping (appropriately, in my opinion) of passionate. Intriguing to me has been the way that these mindsets have morphed over time, particularly over the past 24 years, starting in 2000, when pain was designated as the "5th vital sign" by the Veteran's Health Administration and Congress. Interestingly, that very same year was also designated as the beginning of the *Decade of Pain Control and Research* [1]. It seemed back then as if the gap between the appropriate assessment and treatment for people with pain, acute, malignant, and chronic non-malignant (as it was referred to back then) pain was going to get smaller—significantly smaller, because pain was finally going to get the attention it deserved. This 10-year period was going to be devoted to a concerted effort to answer all the plaguing questions about how pain should be assessed and treated. It was only the second time in U.S. history the Federal Government had declared a "Decade" devoted to any specific disease, medical condition, or organ system. The other instance was in 1990, 10 years earlier when President George Bush declared that year to be the beginning of the *Decade of the Brain* [2]. The thrust of this first "Decade Designation" was multifaceted, hoping to promote attention to and promote research about common diseases affecting the brain including Alzheimer's disease, as well as stroke, schizophrenia, autism, and impairments of speech, language, and hearing. It was also postulated that brain research could help to provide important answers to persistent questions about how to best wage and effective "War on Drugs" and help to provide greater insight into how people become addicted to drugs and other substances and how drugs affect the brain, along with facilitating better development of effective treatments for chemical dependency and to help particularly assist in understanding and preventing the harm done to the unborn children of women who use drugs and alcohol during their pregnancy. Until the writing of this book, I never realized the relationship between these

© The Author(s), under exclusive license to Springer Nature Switzerland AG 2024
K. L. Zacharoff, P. Migdal, *Pain, Drugs, and Ethics*,
https://doi.org/10.1007/978-3-031-63018-7_1

two designated decades, but now see that there were many common and intertwining intentional themes.

I remember thinking it truly seemed as if the 20-year period from late 2000 to 2020 was going to be an exciting time in the field of pain research, and ultimately provide so many answers to challenges facing the medical community and people living with pain in the United States. I remember it all, particularly the year 2000 as a critically important and exciting time for members of what we refer to as the "Pain Community"—those clinicians, organizations, and other interested stakeholders who had dedicated their lives and efforts toward providing much needed care to the millions of people with pain.

As many today look back on the designation of pain as the 5th vital sign, it interesting as to just how much finger-pointing takes place today with respect to why it happened, and many lament the negative impact it has had on our society over the past 24 years. Many passionate individuals argue that this elevation of pain to "vital sign status" was concocted as a marketing strategy by pharmaceutical companies to reinforce increases in prescribing of pain medications (particularly, if not solely manufacturers of opioid analgesics), ultimately throwing fuel onto the fire of what would become a national overdose epidemic. Others blame nonprofit advocacy or quality assessment organizations like the Joint Commission (then referred to by the name The Joint Commission on Accreditation of Healthcare Organizations or JCAHO), a nonprofit organization created in 1951 with the mission "*To continuously improve health care for the public, in collaboration with other stakeholders, by evaluating health care organizations and inspiring them to excel in providing safe and effective care of the highest quality and value*" for making this designation as a result of industry funding and/or lobby influence. Others are suspect of some of the pain medical societies which existed at the time, such as the American Pain Society, The American Academy of Pain Medicine, and the American Pain Foundation to name a few. In many people's opinions, the problem was again rooted in the fact that in many circumstances, a significant amount of funding of these organizations was tainted, because it was provided by industry—pharmaceutical companies, device manufacturers, and other potential sources that could not be rationally considered to be free of conflict of interest, regardless of the "illusion" of the separational barrier between promotional and nonpromotional funding source designations.

My perspective about these controversies as I reflect on them is that people's memories may sometimes tend to be short when it comes to recollecting sequences of events and the circumstances that took place, especially when the perception is that negative consequences resulted. I am not confident that many people who are involved in this debate today were even present or engaged in the pain and substance use landscape in 2000 when these and other events took place and am even less sure that people remember the specific sequence of events leading up to the designation of pain as the 5th vital sign. I don't know if people consider or remember that in the mid-to-late 1990s, that litigation of healthcare professionals (mostly physicians at that time) for undertreating people's pain was not an uncommon occurrence. Successful litigations in many cases, for not giving patients the pain treatment they needed or deserved. I'm don't think many remember a then passionate and vocal lobbying effort by the American Cancer Society to improve the scope and quality of pain assessment and treatment for people with malignant pain, and for that matter people with non-malignant (now referred to as non-cancer) pain. I'm not sure if people remember that when it came to pain, things *needed* to change—for the better.

I think many may also may not remember or know that at this very same point in time, patients were empowered with a *"Pain Care Bill of Rights,"* which considered appropriate pain assessment and treatment to be a basic right for all. This affirmed to patients that they had the right to expect to: (1) have their report of pain taken seriously and to be treated with dignity and respect by doctors, nurses, pharmacists, and other healthcare professionals; (2) have their pain thoroughly assessed and promptly treated; (3) be informed by their healthcare provider about what may be causing their pain, possible treatments, and the benefits, risks, and costs of each; (4) participate actively in decisions about how to manage their pain; (5) have their pain reassessed regularly and the treatment adjusted if their pain had not been eased; (6) be referred to a pain specialist if their pain persisted; and (7) get clear and prompt answers to questions, take time to make decisions, and refuse a particular type of treatment if so desired.

Additionally important, and not often mentioned in the continuing debate today, is that in October 2000, Congress introduced and passed the Bill H.R. 5544, *The Pain Relief Promotion Act of 2000*, which in addition to promoting adequate treatment of pain, contained *"Title II: Use of Controlled Substances Consistent With the Controlled Substances Act"* that amended the Controlled Substances Act of 1970 to underscore that *"alleviating pain or discomfort in the usual course of professional practice is a legitimate medical purpose for the dispensing, distributing, or administering a controlled substance that is consistent with public health and safety, even if it may increase the risk of death."*

Retrospectively, it seems clear that at the time there was an alignment from most if not all involved parties to help people with pain who were in many cases being left untreated, neglected, or even avoided. There was certainly a sense that more research needed to be done to find better pain treatments, and that compassion and empathy for people with pain was very much a missing piece of the healthcare puzzle of the time. Certainly, this alliance included the industry members who stood to substantially benefit from these developments, but to simplistically point to their potential economic gains as the single driving force of this sea change may be somewhat misguided. Virtually every stakeholder, including patient advocacy groups, healthcare professional organizations, pharmaceutical and device manufacturers, regulatory agencies, state medical boards, and politicians were devoted to the idea that improved levels of pain control should be given to the poorly defined but significantly large number of patients who were deemed to have been denied the assessment and satisfactory treatment they were entitled to. And this was a mindset that had significant majority buy-in and momentum. It is important to mention that the above-mentioned initiatives are certainly not a comprehensive list of all engaged parties, but it is a fairly accurate representation of what was happening to help to bring pain "into the limelight" of medical care at the time, with these serving as good representative examples of what the collective thinking was at the time.

So from that point on it seemed as if pain was here to stay, and as a result, patients everywhere would now be queried about whether they were experiencing *any* pain at every clinical encounter, regardless of the reason for the visit, and how they would rate their answer based on (most commonly) a scale of 0–10, with 0 being "no pain at all" and 10 being "pain as bad as it could possibly be." Pain ratings were embedded into virtually every intake and assessment form and considered to be basic information that needed to be documented in the medical record by all, because not unlike heart rate, respiratory rate, blood pressure, and temperature, it was a "vital sign." Other tools were developed to assess pain in children and cognitively impaired and noncommunicative patients; faces expressing smiles or frowns could help estimate a patient's rating of their pain. Patients came to expect to be questioned about whether they were experiencing pain at every clinic visit, armed with an answer and expectations about how their pain would be treated.

The Conundrum of Pain

It didn't take long for what I refer to as "*the conundrum*" associated with all the increased attention to pain to surface in a variety of different ways. First and foremost, how clinicians responded to this widely publicized and omnipresent outcry for better assessment and treatment of pain was relatively consistent across the country and very targeted—with a dramatic increase in the prescriptions written for pain medications (i.e., opioid analgesics) for patient reported complaints of pain. It seemed reasonable to most that not unlike other detected abnormal findings or reported symptoms that once pain was identified and documented in the medical record that something needed to be done about it. Patients had rights, and a documented "significant" pain rating was not only a liability if left ignored, but not in line with accepted medical thinking at the time—a sense of duty to identify and treat—patients had a right to that. The armamentarium for pain treatment was relatively small, and opioid analgesics were front and center as the "go to" choice of treatment for many, if not most instances of reported significant pain. Another contributor to the conundrum was that there were many outstanding unanswered questions about efficacious pain treatments. The research would supposedly be coming, but what to do in the moment was a quandary for many practitioners. Could one conclude which patient-reported pain ratings should be considered "significant" and which not? Was a pain rating of 0–4 not necessarily worthy of treatment, but a 5–10 rating conclusively worthy of treatment? Which patients' ratings merited treatment with an opioid analgesic, and which did not and could be treated with nonopioid? It seems as if the rapid and increased desire to assess and document the presence or absence of pain with a simple numeric rating system resulted in an arbitrary, poorly defined, and inconsistent metric for treatment decision-making across the gamut of nonexpert, frontline practice settings. Even within practice settings, there could be an expectation that there might not be consensus about the threshold for treatment with an opioid analgesic. There was also little agreement about how to measure progress or response to pain treatment when and if an opioid was prescribed. Questions were abundant. Was an improvement in pain rating of 2 points on the 0–10 scale adequate or significant? What about 3 points? Did it matter what the initial pain rating was as a further complicating factor? What was the appropriate course of action if pain was reported to be the same or worse on reassessment? Which increases in pain rating would be thought to be a "failure" of response versus normal variance in a population with respect to how they metabolized opioid medications (e.g., "fast, normal, or slow" metabolizers)? Looking back now, it seems as if the number of increased "unknowns" well outpaced the "knowns," and the desire to help to treat people with pain may have preceded understanding of a concrete, reproducible idea of what constituted a positive pain treatment outcome.

A complicating matter and important theme which will appear many times throughout the course of this book—the fact that there is a unique aspect about pain which in many ways separates it from other common medical conditions; that these patients have a voice and a vote with respect to the determination of what constitutes a successful treatment outcome. This can be somewhat radical thinking even for most healthcare professionals today, in a time of increased focus on patient-centered care and shared medical decision-making is considered paramount. It should not be difficult to imagine the myriad of challenges this notion presented to the medical community some 24 years ago, when the 5th vital sign came into existence. Clinicians had been very much used to the idea of identifying an abnormal finding on history and physical examination, prescribing some course of treatment, and then in a relatively paternalistic way determining on re-assessment whether the goals of that treatment had been reached or not. The idea of including the patient in the decision-making process with respect to an abnormal blood pressure or serum glucose and the appropriate course of treatment might seem laughable to many, but with respect to pain, suddenly patients had a "seat" at the decision-making table, and if they were not satisfied with their pain treatment, then it might not be a case of the patient failing a course of therapy, but *the clinician failing the patient*. This may or may not have been a contributing factor to the relatively low level of consensus about how to assess clinical outcomes of pain treatment at the time, but even under the best circumstances, if clinicians were relatively inconsistent in terms of their thinking about how a patient with a certain pain rating (5–10, for example) should be treated, patients were now further complicating variables in this equation that in many cases clinicians did not have prior experience with or expect at the time.

There are many other factors to be considered with respect to the conundrum of pain, but there is one which I consider to be the most important one of all—a profound, prevalent, and stark absence of education about pain and its management in healthcare professional training programs. Waiting until the end of the *Decade of Pain Control and Research* to provide answers and evidence-based recommendations to healthcare professionals was not an acceptable option. Clinicians were already "in the river," in many cases without the foundational knowledge of how to figure out the best course of action uniformly and consistently when pain was queried for and discovered. It is impossible in hindsight not to label this as a major contributing factor to the increasing number of opioid-related overdoses that started to appear long before it was deemed to be of "epidemic" proportion. Although not well defined in terms of incidence until 2011, in a report titled *Relieving Pain in America: A Blueprint for Transforming Prevention, Care, Education, and Research*" by the Institutes of Medicine (IOM) [3] it became clear, once pain became the 5th vital sign, that millions of people in the United States experienced some type of pain (acute or chronic) at any given time—*millions*. The significance of this newly discovered, seemingly large number of people with pain may be an item of contention for many now, but in the face of a lack of education, availability of reproducible assessment tools, and poor or completely absent level of consensus about what to do for these patients confounded many and may have further contributed to what is now referred to as the period of liberal prescribing of opioid analgesics to treat pain.

Attempts to help to fill the glaring educational gaps presented themselves in concert with the vital sign designation of pain. In many cases, educational programs were created and made available by pharmaceutical companies that were in the business of manufacturing and marketing opioid analgesics, not developed by the "promotional side" of these companies, but by their "nonpromotional" teams. "Firewalls" existed to specifically prevent the corruption of nonpromotional educational programs with promotional messaging. To be successfully accredited for CME/CE, proof of this separation would need to be provided to the accrediting organization. In many cases, these initiatives took the form of continuing medical education (CME or CE) programs, which allowed them to serve a dual purpose: to participate in and acquire the mandatory number of CME/CE credits required to renew license registrations, and to get the much-needed education about how to best assess patients with pain safely and effectively. In fact, in certain situations, providing a detailed framework of educational programs to the U.S. Food and Drug Administration (FDA) called RiskMAPs (Risk Minimization Action Plans) was considered part and parcel of many FDA drug applications and approval processes for many medications, including prescription pain medications such as opioids. Industry-based educational programs helped to provide education, tools which could be used in clinical practice, and in some cases included treatment algorithms. All with the intention of helping to fill educational gaps that existed surrounding pain management in all but the most expert level of clinical practice settings. Publication plans for pharmaceutical companies and device manufacturers were deemed (and still are today) to be critical components of part of the process of doing business, the result being generation of peer-reviewed publications that would complement the educational process, in many cases written by thought leaders who were well known in the expert level field of pain management. All with the intention of helping to answer the questions and fill the educational divide to those on the front line.

Topics beyond the scope of this book include the potential ethical questions raised by these types of industry-funded educational tactics and strategies, the possibility of conflict of interest, subliminal marketing messaging, etc. They are in and of themselves topics of many debates which take place today regarding CME/CE programs for any variety of therapies, regardless of the medical condition, but very passionate due to the increasing number of annual drug-related fatalities. The point being made is that there was a desire for knowledge about pain, and there were numerous attempts to help to feed that hunger. Independent, nonindustry funded, unbiased academic avenues of education did not seem to present themselves plentifully in the 10 years of the *Decade of Pain Control and Research* (2000–2010). That was and still is problematic on many levels.

The Conundrum of Pain Education

It is unclear as to whether healthcare training programs, such as medical schools, were so entrenched in competition for the space in their curricula, or they just did not consider pain education to be relevant at the time, but in many cases, pain was glaringly missing, along with education about assessment and treatment of substance use disorders and addiction. One might think that the push to improve pain control and the need to increase awareness about the potential dangers associated with indiscriminate prescribing of opioids would have ensured that these topics found their way into the curriculum of training programs relatively quickly. As Mezei et al. [4] pointed out in their 2011 publication of their analysis of pain education in North American medical schools, *"although pain education was identified in 1988 as an important remedy for the undertreatment of pain, progress toward effective programs that educate future clinicians has been slow. While all allied health professionals need education about pain, deficiencies are conspicuous in medical education."* Concluding their analysis to show that *"in short, pain education was limited and fragmentary."*

As someone who considers the education of our future healthcare professionals to be a critical component of a long-term solution to both the safe and effective treatment of patients with pain and the overdose epidemic we experience in the United States today [5], it was disheartening and oxymoronic for me and others that the *Decade of Pain Control and Research* had come and gone without firmly entrenching education about pain and substance use disorders into medical school curriculums around the country. It seemed confounding that elevation of pain rating to vital sign status, pain being one of the most common reasons that people seek medical attention, coupled with the worrisome concordance of increased opioid prescribing and overdose deaths were not enough to create the impetus for education for about these topics to become part of core training.

It was in approximately 2004 that I became interested in earnest about the need to educate the clinicians already in practice that I felt truly needed the education the most—nonexpert frontline practitioners. The "Pain Community" had its regional and annual meetings to discuss new and old developments about how best to treat pain, but it seemed to me that there was very little to no broad communication about new and foundational topics of pain education. Many important papers were being published in pain journals, but not in mainstream medical journals. Here we were almost at the mid-point of the *Decade of Pain Control and Research*, and the education was not flowing to the clinicians on whose shoulders pain treatment most often rested upon—primary care clinicians. I decided to devote my future efforts to help be a bridge across that educational gap. I firmly believed that with most opioid analgesic prescriptions being written by these practitioners, it was a key ingredient to mitigating the conundrum.

By 2011, the *Decade of Pain Control and Research* was over, and it seemed clear that healthcare professional education at all levels was crucial to a better path forward. Unfortunately, that did not happen in any significant way. Industry-sponsored CME/CE programs continued to be the most widely available form of pain education, along with sparse sessions at large frontline practitioner's conferences about the basics. A commentary in *Pain Medicine News* by Dr. Andrea Trescot (then President of the American Society of Interventional Pain Physicians) in 2008 titled *Frontline Failure: PCPs Often Unarmed Against Pain* aptly summarized the state of pain education at the time. It resonated with me very much. Dr. Trescot stated that education had not reached "soldiers in the trenches," primary care physicians (PCPs), who are typically the clinicians called upon to see patients with pain. Dr. Trescot urged that education needed to start with residency program-level education for future physicians in practice. The commentary also stressed that in addition to addressing educational deficits, better rapport between PCPs and Pain Specialists needed to exist, comparable to the way PCPs communicate with specialists about other medical conditions (e.g., cardiologists when coronary artery disease is being treated). Dr. Trescot concluded better education of PCPs was important to our ability to provide appropriate treatment for patients suffering from pain and associated disability. Something that will be discussed later in this text are the dilemmas involving the use of opioid analgesics to treat pain (Chap. 7). But it is important to mention here that also in 2011 the Office of National Drug Control Policy (ONDCP), an agency of the White House which coordinates the nation's drug policies, declared the number of overdose deaths related to prescription opioids to be of "epidemic" proportions. The *"Opioid Epidemic"* was born.

A report was published by ONDCP outlining a plan focused on combating the abuse of prescription drugs titled *Epidemic: Responding to America's Prescription Drug Abuse Crisis* [6]. Four major pillars of this plan were**: (1) education of the public and healthcare providers**, (2) increased utilization of state-run databases (**Prescription Drug Monitoring Programs or PDMPs**) for tracking and monitoring, (3) development of **easily accessible drug disposal programs**, and (4) providing **law enforcement** agencies the support they needed to eradicate "pill mills" and "doctor shoppers." Here is an excerpt from this report about the importance of healthcare professional education:

> *"...prescribers and dispensers, including physicians, physician's assistants, nurse practitioners, pharmacists, nurses, prescribing psychologists, and dentists, all have a role to play in reducing prescription drug misuse and abuse. Most receive little training on the importance of appropriate prescribing and dispensing of opioids to prevent adverse effects, diversion, and addiction. Outside of specialty addiction treatment programs, most healthcare providers have received minimal training in how to recognize substance abuse in their patients. Most medical, dental, pharmacy, and other health professional schools do not*

provide in-depth training on substance abuse; often, substance abuse education is limited to classroom or clinical electives. Moreover, students in these schools may only receive limited training on treating pain.

A national survey of medical residency programs in 2000 found that of the programs studied, only 56 percent required substance use disorder training, and the number of curricular hours in the required programs varied between 3 and 12 hours. A 2008 follow-up survey found that some progress has been made to improve medical school, residency, and post-residency substance abuse education; however, these efforts have not been uniformly applied in all residency programs or medical schools.

***Educating prescribers on substance abuse is critically important,** because even brief interventions by primary care providers have proven effective in reducing or eliminating substance abuse in people who abuse drugs but are not yet addicted to them. In addition, educating healthcare providers about prescription drug abuse will promote awareness of this growing problem among prescribers so they will not over-prescribe the medication necessary to treat minor conditions. This, in turn, will reduce the amount of unused medication sitting in medicine cabinets in homes across the country."*

The following action items detailed in this plan included:

- **Working with Congress to amend Federal law** to require practitioners (such as physicians, dentists, and others authorized to prescribe) who request DEA registration to prescribe controlled substances to be t**rained on responsible opioid prescribing practices as a precondition of registration**. This training would include assessing and addressing signs of abuse and/or dependence.
- **Requiring drug manufacturers**, through the Opioid Risk Evaluation and Mitigation Strategy (REMS), **to develop effective educational materials and initiatives to train practitioners** on the appropriate use of opioid pain relievers.
- Federal agencies that support their own healthcare **systems increasing continuing education for their practitioners and other healthcare providers on proper prescribing and disposal of prescription drugs**.
- **Working with appropriate medical and healthcare boards to encourage them to require education curricula in health professional schools** (medical, nursing, pharmacy, and dental) and continuing education programs to include instruction on the safe and appropriate use of opioids to treat pain while minimizing the risk of addiction and substance abuse. Additionally, work with relevant medical, nursing, dental, and pharmacy student groups to help disseminate educational materials, and establish student programs that can give community educational presentations on prescription drug abuse and substance abuse.

Ironically, it is still not uncommon today, 24 years after the 5th vital sign designation, that many future Primary Care and other physicians may proceed throughout the course of their medical school and residency education with little to virtually no education about pain and its management. It may be even less likely that related topics such as substance use disorders and addiction are covered for all but the most specialized medical specialties. As the *Decade of Pain Control and Research* moved further and further away in our nation's rear-view mirror, it became clear that relatively few of its goals were achieved. Expert knowledge and scientifically derived evidence-based information was not successfully identified and translated to those who needed it most. In many people's opinions, including patients with pain, the overall state of pain management is possibly worse today than it had been before the "*Decade*" began.

Education is not something that has completely evaded stakeholder discussion and debate. In fact, regulatory agencies such as the Drug Enforcement Administration (DEA), the Food and Drug Administration (FDA), and the Federation of State Medical Boards (FSMB) deliberated and explored methods to provide pain education to clinicians. Most of these educational efforts have been focused on safe and effective opioid prescribing and have been voluntary in nature. While the programs developed have been well-intentioned, barriers have included the challenge of getting clinicians to donate their precious time to participate. When the subject of making education mandatory is brought up, pushback has been significant and quite vocal about the potential resource-related hardships related to that route of delivery. However, many State Medical Boards across the country have implemented mandatory requirements which are often a condition of maintenance of licensure to include a portion of required continuing medical education devoted to pain, opioid prescribing, substance use etc. In most cases, the requirement is approximately 3 credit hours of education about these topics every year or typical registration renewal period, and it is not difficult to surmise that this barely scratches the surface of the education needed.

In 2011, the FDA mandated *Risk Evaluation and Risk Mitigation Strategies (REMS)* first for extended- release/long-acting (ER/LA) opioid analgesics, a key component of the REMS was "elements to assure safe use" (ETASU) including education of prescribers [7]. In fact, this REMS included what was called the *FDA Blueprint for Prescriber Education for Extended-Release and Long-Acting Opioid Analgesics*. This blueprint was quite detailed and had the potential to provide a significant amount of education to clinicians treating patients with pain and weigh the risks and benefits of pain treatment with ER/LA opioid medications. Numerous concerns existed about this approach to filling the educational void. First, this education was going to be funded by a collective consisting of the opioid manufacturers; some posited that this would be just another form of industry-funded educational efforts with subliminal messages. Second, this education would be voluntary, and the ability to prescribe ER/LA opioids was not conditional on completing the REMS education program. It was unclear to many how to engage clinicians and entice them to take advantage of the education if it was not conditional to a requirement in some way. Third, there were a tremendous number of ER/LA opioid REMS education programs that became available, that although they did follow the "educational blueprint", varied from one another significantly. This created confusion for individuals interested in obtaining education, as it wasn't perfectly clear as to redundancy or distinguishing characteristics of the various REMS education programs available. In many ways, these programs were competing by trying to meet metrics like number of prescribers completing the programs, etc. to continue to be funded. Lastly (but not comprehensively), many didn't understand why the REMS education at that time only applied to ER/LA opioids and not all formulations of opioid analgesics, which led to further confusion.

In 2018, the FDA expanded the REMS to include all opioid analgesics, with an updated educational blueprint. Once again, many questions existed regarding whether someone who did participate in the initial REMS education should then go through it again.

Ethical Perspectives

The past 24 years have been a turbulent time in the pain management community for clinicians, other stakeholders (most notably regulators), and, most importantly, people with pain. As we have reviewed in this chapter, efforts intended to create a greater sense of advocacy and treatment for patients with pain have been met with high levels of reactivity blended with equal doses of controversy.

Passionate and heated debates continue today on a variety of levels. Nothing happens in a vacuum, and this subject is certainly no different. The overdose epidemic alone has made navigating a path forward which maintains access to opioid medications for appropriate patients but mitigates societal risk from overdose fatalities somewhere between difficult to near impossible to achieve. Many seek to retract pain's designation as the 5th vital sign, with the sentiment it may have done more harm than good. Research has not provided sufficient answers to outstanding questions about long-term efficacious treatment of people with chronic pain, and barriers which had been removed seem to be resurfacing. At the height of pain treatment advocacy, the distinction between cancer-related (then referred to as malignant pain) pain and noncancer-related pain (then referred to as nonmalignant pain) seemed to dissolve. This delineation seems to be alive and well today. It is not uncommon for there to be a sense that someone with cancer-related pain is more entitled to opioid treatment than someone with noncancer pain, particularly if there is no identifiable cause or diagnosis associated with it. A separate set of "rules" can set the stage for confusion, further fueling the conundrum. Unquestionably, there is an emotional component to this mindset, but it can be a very slippery slope toward depriving someone of compassionate, empathetic, and ethical pain treatment because they might not merit an emotional benefit of the doubt. If the presence or absence of cancer becomes an attribute by which someone can be given or denied treatment, the stage can be set for bias, stigma, prejudice, and disparate pain treatment to exist.

Let's remember that all of this has been happening in the absence of adequate education to prepare healthcare professionals to effectively grapple with these complicated, nuanced issues. I have heard experts that I have the utmost respect for discouragingly say that in their opinion "*education doesn't make a difference.*" In my opinion, if we believe that, then all might be lost. Virtually every fiber in the fabric of medical education is devoted to increasing knowledge and capitalizing on it to improve the quality of care provided. We need to identify the knowledge gaps, eradicate them for our future clinicians, and collectively try to be less reactive to the "*pendulum swings*" that impose themselves and impact the way we approach our patients, and ground ourselves with the aspiration to provide the most ethical care to patients with pain that we can—because **there is no such thing as an "ethical pendulum."**

References

1. Brennan F. The US congressional "decade on pain control and research" 2001–2011: a review. J Pain Palliat Care Pharmacother. 2015;29:212–27.
2. George Bush, President of the United States. Presidential Proclamation 6158. July 18, 1990.
3. IOM (Institute of Medicine). Relieving pain in America: a blueprint for transforming prevention, care, education, and research. Washington, DC: The National Academies Press; 2011.
4. Mezei L, Murinson BB. Johns Hopkins pain curriculum development team. Pain education in north American medical schools. J Pain. 2011;12:1199–208.
5. Briggs E. Evaluating the impact of pain education: how do we know we have made a difference? Br J Pain. 2012;6(2):85–91.
6. Office of National Drug Control Policy, Washington, DC 20500, United States. Epidemic: responding to America's prescription drug abuse crisis. NCJ Number 234164. April 2011.
7. Opioid Analgesic Risk Evaluation and Mitigation Strategy (REMS) that is required by the U.S. Food and Drug Administration (FDA). https://opioidanalgesicrems.com/home.html. Accessed 16 June 2023.

Pain as a Disease

2

Pain Defined

Except for those people with the rare condition known as congenital insensitivity to pain (CIP), pain is a something that virtually all of us have experienced at one or many times in our lives. But it is important to remember that pain is somewhat of a "black box," in that only the sufferer fully understands the experience. Pain has both subjective and objective components, the proportions of which may be variable, all of which must be given consideration and treated. Additionally, attention must be paid to the temporal nature of the pain, as treatment strategies for *acute pain* may differ dramatically from those for *chronic pain*.

At its most basic level, pain functions most often as a protective mechanism that quickly sends signals to the brain that our body is in physical danger and generally elicits some kind of rapid response. In the absence of an expected pain-provoking situation like surgery, most of us think of pain as an *adaptive* safety mechanism that warns us about further harm. For example, if we touch a hot stove, we feel a burning type of pain, and pull away to prevent further harm from it. In this situation, *pain protects us*. While pain is a ubiquitous phenomenon, it is not uncommon that it varies from person to person. The same set of circumstances can cause significant pain in one individual, and little or none in another. The reason that pain in this context is considered adaptive is because it is possible that over time our bodies can "overcome" the pain associated with certain stimuli and become "trained," ultimately leading to a decrease in the painful experience. Very often, this involves our minds—something we will cover a bit later in this chapter. It is also important to keep in mind that it is possible in other situations that pain can be or become *maladaptive*; meaning that even in the absence of a painful stimulus, one still experiences pain. A common example of this would be phantom limb pain, where someone experiences pain in an arm, leg, or other body part that has been amputated, and for some reason the person continues to perceive pain as if were in the absent body part. In many contexts, it is reasonable to think about pain most commonly as being a purely neurologic event, explained and resulting solely through nervous system activity.

© The Author(s), under exclusive license to Springer Nature Switzerland AG 2024
K. L. Zacharoff, P. Migdal, *Pain, Drugs, and Ethics*,
https://doi.org/10.1007/978-3-031-63018-7_2

However, pain is actually a number of complex processes that not only involve the nervous system, but also involve our psychology. Pain is much more than a physiologic phenomenon, it is *an experience*, If you think about experiences in your life, you likely are thinking about memories, feelings, and emotions. All of these are important things to consider related to the pain experience.

Briefly, nociceptive pain, or pain related to a painful stimulus like the example mentioned above involves a number of neurologic phenomena in order for it to occur. In simple terms and under normal circumstances, first a painful stimulus (such as a pinprick) is "translated" or *transduced* into a signal or impulse that will travel through the nerves at or near the point of stimulation. Once the nervous impulse exists, it travels or is *transmitted* toward the spinal cord to be sent upward toward the brain. Our nervous systems have the remarkable capacity to *modulate* or modify strength and speed of transmission of the signal which can result in an increase or decrease in pain intensity. This means that in some cases, the signal might be dampened, and in others might be amplified. This depends on the individual circumstances related to the painful stimulus and other things that may be happening at the same time or have happened prior to the stimulus. Once the signals reach the brain, they are *perceived*. The brain now is "aware" of the pain and may or may not interpret the signal to respond in some way, whether it be a physical action (like pulling the hand away from the source of the pain), a physiologic response (like releasing adrenaline), or both. At a neurologic level, it is fair to say that there is a high level of predictive nature of transduction, transmission, and modulation under normal situations. At the point of perception though, there can be a high level of variability, and this is where pain becomes an experience, one that can be highly subjective in nature. Something else to consider is the fact that perception of pain by the brain and the reflexive subsequent responses do not necessarily require a conscious state. This means that someone in a semi or even unconscious state may still elicit physiologic responses to pain, such as an elevated heart rate, blood pressure, respiratory rate, etc. The typical conscious reactions to pain such as crying, grimacing, and moaning may be absent, but the pain is still present. This simplified pathophysiologic explanation of nociceptive pain is intended to help illustrate how pain is often very narrowly defined by many, with pain resulting from a purely ***mechanistic*** and ***neurophysiologic*** perspective. In fact, there have been many experts over the past 20 or so years who have promoted the idea that the best way to treat pain is to identify the mechanisms involved and to target them.

While the pain pathways mentioned above *are* important to consider when we think about pain assessment and treatment planning, these constructs most often apply to how we approach most types of **acute pain**. Acute pain is usually the result of an injury or illness that is time-limited in nature and designated based on temporal classification, most often recent onset, and lasting 1 month or less. Low back pain after an injury, acute headache, and postoperative pain are examples of acute pain. Acute pain is generally thought to have the biologic function of alerting the individual to harm and preparing for the "fight-or-flight" response to danger as mentioned above. It is an important component of the vital, protective "sentry system" that permits us to live in an environment filled with potential dangers. Diagnosing and treating the underlying cause of pain, in addition to treating the symptomatic pain, are the critical elements of pain management. The lack of education of clinicians often leaves them unprepared to approach pain assessment in any other way than to treat it as if the pain were acute, mechanistic pain. Measures taken may often be reductionistic in nature with the intention of investigating and treating the underlying cause and reducing a self-reported pain rating (0–10). Most commonly, this also involves using pharmacologic agents, utilizing a purely **biomedical approach**. This may not be the best course(s) of action when treating subacute or chronic pain, where much more may be taking place. Additionally, this does not consider the *neuropsychological* and *humanistic* perspectives of pain which are reflective of the important role of the biopsychosocial model of pain treatment.

Subacute pain is pain that persists beyond the 1-month duration of acute pain, and is usually attributed to a slower rate of healing from a known injury, etc. Often occupying the space in time between acute and chronic pain (1 month to 3 months), although not often considered by many, subacute pain is likely *the most important indicator* of likelihood or presence of risk factors for someone transitioning from a short-lived, acute painful condition to a more persistent and maladaptive one. Comprehensive assessment and efficacious treatment of subacute pain may likely be the most important steps that can be taken to mitigate long-term pain, but in the face of educational deficits, many clinicians may approach this type of pain no differently than acute pain—with increasing doses of medications, and the goal of reducing pain ratings.

Chronic pain is pain that persists and does not resolve spontaneously. Often arbitrarily defined as pain that persists for 3 months duration or longer, chronic pain often lasts beyond the period of expected healing, or after healing has taken place. Patients with a chronic pain complaint may have no evidence of pathology or identifiable cause of pain on presentation, and onset of pain and descriptors may also be unclear. These attributes may sometimes contribute to questioning of the veracity of pain-related complaints of this type, further complicating and sometimes even biasing the clinician's overall impressions. The assessment of chronic pain requires more attention to the biopsychosocial aspects of the patient in the context of their pain-related complaints, and likely more focus on those aspects when it comes to treatment planning as well. A reductionistic approach that targets a "cure" for pain is significantly less likely to succeed when treating patients with chronic pain.

If defining pain was a simple case of temporal classification, there might be more consensus about its treatment. However, pain is not that simple, and this often becomes a very significant and often confounding issue for patients with pain-related complaints. As strange as it sounds, **how clinicians define pain can vary widely** and may often be inconsistent in nature. Clinically, this can lead to inconsistencies in how pain is assessed and, more importantly, effectively treated. Although it might seem as if all healthcare professionals define pain in a uniform way, in many cases they do not. In fact, there has been such a wide variation about how pain is defined that the International Association for the Study of Pain (IASP) was compelled to define and then redefine pain twice over the past 45 years in an attempt to achieve greater consensus and consistency, first in 1979 and most recently in 2020.

The IASP is the leading independent global organization dedicated to "bringing together scientists, clinicians, healthcare professionals, and policymakers from around the world with the mission of bringing relief to those in pain" [1]. How we define pain is so important is because how we define it will likely impact everything that we do to help patients and trying to treat it.

In 1979, the IASP recognized the dilemmas created by the existence of differing definitions of pain, and after careful deliberation released a definition of pain that was intended to create global consensus of how pain was defined. The IASP in progressive fashion proposed that clinicians needed to consider that pain was more than just a simple neurological phenomenon. This definition [2] stated that pain was "*An unpleasant sensory and emotional experience associated with actual or potential tissue damage or described in terms of such damage.*" This highlighted the notion that pain might exist in the absence of evidence of tissue damage (potential tissue damage), but retrospectively did not have much clinical impact. This was partly because the majority of clinicians did not know how to interpret it or consider how to treat pain occurring in the absence of obvious tissue damage. Once again, there was the burden of a requirement for *belief*; the belief that pain could exist in the absence of measurable physical evidence to support its presence. However, this definition of pain was a significant and groundbreaking advancement because it considered what is mentioned at the beginning of this chapter, that pain was **not only a sensory experience**, but also could be an **emotional** one. Despite many subsequently criticizing the IASP for not considering the inclusion of more detail about the cognitive and social aspects of pain, at least the proposal that pain could solely be an emotional experience opened the door for it to be considered as something more than just a sequence of neurological pathways.

The idea that pain can also be an emotional experience is obvious to most. That someone could "feel" pain resulting from other sources than a physical painful stimulus, such as from suffering a loss, experiencing some kind of emotional trauma, or a variety of nonsensory, psychologically initiated reasons does not seem unreasonable. It seems as if this should have been obvious to most clinicians and other important stakeholders (such as regulatory agencies, politicians, etc.) in 1979, but it was not. In fact, 21 years later in 2000 when pain was designated the 5th vital sign, clinicians were instructed to query patients about their pain ratings on a scale of 0–10, with the emphasis placed on assessment of **physical pain**, and **not emotional pain**. Educational deficits and lack of dissemination about the 1979 definition of pain likely contributed to this lack of awareness about these different dimensions of pain.

To give some perspective, in 2011, when the IOM report previously mentioned in Chap. 1 was published, it was estimated that there were approximately 100 million people in the U.S. suffering from pain at any given time. There were approximately five thousand Board-Certified Pain Specialists at the time. This translated to (and still translates to today) the majority of patients with pain-related complaints being assessed and managed by frontline practitioners like those in Family Medicine and Internal Medicine, with most of these clinicians having received little or no education on the subject of pain during the course of their medical training. In summary, twenty years after the IASP attempted to bring consensus to the way pain was defined, pain was designated the 5th vital sign in the United States, and the *Decade of Pain Control and Research* began in 2000.

In July 2020 the members of the IASP felt compelled to redefine pain once again, [3] responding to the lack of progress that had been made in how pain was assessed and treated globally. The intention was stated that this updated definition of pain was "*to better convey the nuances and the complexity of pain and the hope that it would lead to improved assessment and management of those with pain*." The IASP received input from a multitude of stakeholders in the development process which was novel; it included both people with pain and their caregivers. This revised definition described pain as "*An **unpleasant sensory and emotional experience** associated with, or resembling that associated with, actual or potential tissue damage*." My first impression of this new definition was that it was not significantly different than the definition put forth in 1979, and if anything, might seem a bit confusing to many. Phrases like "associated with" and "or resembling that associated" resonated with me as legal wording. What did very much make a significant impression on me was the addition of **six qualifying "key notes"** which were intended to complement and fortify the redefinition. It is here that I think the most meaningful changes in the new definition of pain reside. In my opinion, this was groundbreaking because for the first time a significant amount of attention was paid to the other aspects of pain that went far beyond just a numerical pain rating.

The qualifying notes are as follows:

- Pain is always a personal experience that is influenced to varying degrees by biological, psychological, and social factors
- Pain and nociception are different phenomena. Pain cannot be inferred solely from activity in sensory neurons
- Through their life experiences, individuals learn the concept of pain
- A person's report of an experience as pain should be respected
- Although pain usually serves an adaptive role, it may have adverse effects on function and social and psychological well-being
- Verbal description is only one of several behaviors to express pain; inability to communicate does not negate the possibility that a human or a nonhuman animal experiences pain

Considering that pain is *always a personal experience* which is influenced to varying degrees by biological, psychological, and social factors means that as clinicians we need to consider that no two individuals with a pain-related complaint (or diagnosis) will be identical because it is indeed a personal experience. This means that it will also be unlikely that individualized treatment plans will ever be exactly the same for any two individuals as well. In addition to physical findings and pathophysiology, many variables and factors affect the pain experience including personal stressors, social narratives, and support systems and contribute to what is ultimately a unique and personal pain experience.

That *pain and nociception are different phenomena* is a critical point because this implies that we cannot infer pain to result solely from what we explain based on neurological explanations. This means that purely mechanistic explanations of pain do not solely construct the clinical presentation. It also follows that simply asking someone to rate their pain on a scale of 0–10 is not a comprehensive pain assessment. If clinicians consider that these phenomena differ, then the assessment must include gathering information about both.

The idea that individuals *learn the concept of pain* through life experiences means that this information should be part of the foundation of the pain assessment. Inquiring about how pain impacted family and household members during childhood years and even in the patient's past experiences likely have significant value in assessment and treatment planning. Determining parental, guardian, or even sibling behaviors with respect to how pain impacted life and was perceived by the patients social and family circle during formative years could be highly valuable. To consider that people "learn" acceptable responses to pain makes sense, but often may be overlooked. Certainly, there are cultural differences in the way some people react and respond to pain which illustrate this concept.

That *someone's report of pain should be respected* is a requisite part of the ethical delivery of medical care. I think the motivation of the IASP task force was to promote this idea in a qualifying note to underscore the recommendation that we approach patients with a pain-related complaint with a sense of belief as opposed to disbelief.

While pain serves as a protective mechanism, if prolonged, it may have *adverse effects on function and social and psychological well-being.* This means that something our body does to adapt to or protect us can ultimately have negative consequences on our ability to function, to cope and to perform our daily physical and social activities. The reason this is significant is that it implies that a comprehensive pain assessment should capture more information than a subjective rating of pain on a scale of 0–10. Identifying the impact that pain has on physical function, social interactions, and psychological function is more likely to identify more successfully intended or even necessary outcomes of treatment.

It is not uncommon for us to consider the most effective way for someone to communicate their level of pain to be verbally. However, there may be many situations where people with pain lack the capacity to do so. Young children who have not yet learned to talk and older people with varying degrees of cognitive impairment or other issues preventing verbal communication are just two examples of types of patients who commonly may experience pain but do not have the ability to verbally express it. This enforces the notion that **verbal description is only one of many *behaviors* that individuals have to express that they are experiencing pain**, and that we need to be attuned to those behaviors to have the ability to perform a pain assessment in those patient populations as effectively as we would with anyone else.

This revised definition attempts to fill several gaps and misunderstandings about pain, its assessment, and treatment, but is important to note that there were instances of criticism of it. Many found the definition to continue to be somewhat cumbersome in its verbiage and could have been simpler in its wording to facilitate more practical clinical application. Other comments included that there should have been more attention paid to the personal nature of the experience of pain, and reinforcement of gauging its overall impact on quality of life as a metric, acknowledging its subjective nature. Comments like these notwithstanding, it is reasonable to think that if there was a consistent application of this definition of pain incorporated into clinical practices, there could potentially be a significant improvement in the delivery and quality of pain care. By increasing comprehension, this definition of pain could also help to bring down the invisible barrier that exists between the biomedical and biopsychosocial approaches to pain.

Unfortunately, as of this writing, dissemination and subsequent uptake of this revised definition has been poor and, in many cases, nonexistent. Once again, lack of communication and education seems to be a significant hindrance to attempts to improve the care of people in pain. One would think that given the prevalence of pain and the spotlight on the overdose epidemic that this new definition would have been incorporated into every medical school curriculum, every training program for pain specialists, and every continuing education program for frontline practitioners. At a minimum, one might have expected that every pain clinic would have embraced and adopted this new definition of how people with pain are assessed and treated. Disappointingly, other than publishing an article about the revised definition in the IASP's own publication *PAIN*, along with an article about the challenges and barriers that this new definition might face [2] thus far it has not been widely disseminated in mainstream publications such as the *Journal of the American Medical Association*, the *New England Journal of Medicine*, the *Annals of Internal Medicine*, etc. But it has not. In fact, in a recent discussion I had with the Director of a very well-respected Pain Clinic in a large academic center, when queried about the impact the new definition of pain was having on clinical practices in their pain clinic drew the response "*What* new definition?"

Why Pain Is Different

People often use pain as a qualifier of overall quality of life. It seems natural to think that at the final stages of someone's life, successful mitigation of pain and associated suffering would be what anyone would want. Under these circumstances, there is no stigma attached to this pain, no questioning about how severe the pain is, no mention of malingering behavior in the context of the pain, and no doubt cast on whether the pain even exists or not. By most assessments, *comfortable* is the opposite of *painful*, and the capacity to measure comfort or pain in end-of-life situations is not complex, challenging, or subjective. This translates that to make someone comfortable at the end of life is to mitigate their pain. There is no lack of clarity, and nothing is foreign or bewildering to virtually any of us. It is highly unlikely that in one way or another we have not witnessed or experienced this desire for comfort and alleviation of pain for someone at least once in our lives, if not multiple times. An abundance of compassion for someone at the end stages of life leads us to a point where we are somehow willing to forego the subjective nature of pain to alleviate it, personally or professionally. In this situation, we are fully willing to treat something unlike other "vital signs" that cannot be measured with a device like a sphygmomanometer, thermometer, or stethoscope. Something which has no "normal range" or numerical value. Something about pain in this context makes us believe (or suspend belief) that we are doing something morally and ethically good by helping to diminish someone's pain. It seems as if being able to affirm that someone *"didn't suffer,"* *"is not suffering,"* or *"wasn't in pain"* helps us grapple with sadness, sorrow, or impressions about the quality of life or the quality of end of life. All these thoughts, emotions, and feelings are defined by pain and its associated suffering. There is little confusion, wavering, or debate about the relationship between pain and suffering and the desire to treat it to the best of our capabilities.

However, if we consider pain and suffering outside of the above-mentioned context, in the course of everyday life, for example, it seems as if everything changes. In this context, pain becomes something that we cannot practically and objectively measure, that we cannot see, that we cannot test for, and that is challenging for us to confirm, assess, and treat. In this context, pain becomes something which requires belief on our part as clinicians, regulators, law enforcement officials, caretakers, or other stakeholders. Pain now becomes something that needs to be proven to exist. Many question why the United States seems to have an overwhelming preponderance of people with pain. Statements like *"I don't remember people in my grandparent's generation complaining about pain or certainly seeking treatment for it"* are commonly made. For many, pain becomes a "symptom" we wish we never inquired about because in many cases, we were not taught about what to do to treat it once we believe that it exists, or how to believe it exists without stigma, bias, or precognitive thinking. Situationally, the virtuous compassion mentioned above and the sense of duty to alleviate pain suffering and improve quality of life vaporizes based on the context of the individual with a pain-related complaint.

Numerous questions are part of the traditional assessment for people with a pain-related complaint. Is the pain **acute**? Is it **chronic**? What is its **duration**, its **location**, and its **quality**? How does one *rate it* on a scale of 0–10, with 0 being no pain at all, and 10 being pain as bad as it can be? Which face on the diagram most closely aligns with **how you feel** because of your pain? **How** did the pain happen? These are all standard points of information that need to be documented in the medical record. *Rarely* is there an inquiry about how much one *feels they are suffering* due to the pain they are experiencing. What impact pain has on their individual lives. To that point, students or attendees of pain conferences who do receive pain education are often taught that some of the most important questions to ask people with pain are the ones which help to identify the degree to which pain prevents them from functioning in the context of their individual lives. This **functional context** is personal, unique to the individual, and considers not only physical level of function, but also social and psychological level of function as well.

As mentioned in Chapter I, educational deficits have left large gaps for practicing and future healthcare professionals with respect to how to consistently assess patients with a complaint of pain and approach pain beyond capturing a cursory pain rating (stemming from its designated 5th vital sign status). Healthcare professionals typically recommend and implement treatment choices with which they are comfortable. In some cases, the result may be to lead clinicians to avoid seeing or treating patients with a pain-related complaint because their educational foundation has not prepared them adequately to do so.

A 2016 opinion piece published in the *Journal of the American Medical Association* [5] by Dr. Jonathan H. Chen titled "The Patient You Least Want to See" is a compelling example which illustrates the impact of educational deficiencies in clinical training and practice. The author sheds light on how pain and its treatment is often viewed differently from other medical conditions and how future clinicians may often feel unprepared to treat patients with pain, leading them to want to avoid these patients. Writing about his experiences as an intern, Dr. Chen describes being called upon to treat patients with a variety of medical conditions, including pain. He refers to patients with pain as the patient that "*you least want to see*" for a variety of reasons. He details stark differences which existed in his training institution when being called upon to treat patients with pain and write orders for opioid medications, and contrasts these with ordering medications for other medical conditions. He describes being given clear guidance from pharmacists and attending physicians about dosing and the presence of numerous systems checks in place for ordering medications like insulin, potassium, vasopressors, and antibiotics. Alternatively, he related that when it came time to ordering intravenous opioid analgesics for pain, there were "*no questions asked.*" He found the patients he "least wanted to see" were those requesting opioids, reporting that he found himself between challenging pain patients and "*inconsistent supervising Physicians, between the power to prescribe potent medications [like opioids] and learning to compassionately manage pain.*" Discussing the importance of role modeling on trainees' future careers, he reported a dramatic lack of consistency among his teachers that often resulted in "*team splitting and undermined decisions*" when it came to treating pain, especially if opioid medications were involved. He reflected that "*perhaps some find it simpler...to respond to such patients by avoiding them.*" Labeling patients as drug-seekers was a common occurrence. He concludes by expressing his hope that there could be a way to learn and teach a thoughtful, consistent approach to prescribing opioid analgesics for patients with pain in acute inpatient and chronic outpatient settings, not unlike those used for treating other chronic diseases like diabetes. That "*the patient you least want to see is probably the one who needs you the most.*"

Unfortunately, not much has changed since Dr. Chen's opinion piece was published back in 2016. There are several possible explanations for this. One of them being that pain does not often occur in a vacuum, as will be discussed later in this book. Another is the fact that the overdose epidemic is tightly interwoven into the fabric of pain management in our country and complicates and confounds the moral and ethical imperatives to alleviate pain and suffering. However, even though pain is one of the most common reasons that people seek medical attention in the United States, the fact that many training institutions do not have pain assessment and treatment as part of their required core curricula is somewhat of an oxymoron. Considering the overdose epidemic plaguing our nation today, the fact that substance use disorder and addiction is even less likely to be covered as part of basic clinical education borders on baffling to many. If education about hypertension, cardiovascular disease, and diabetes were not comprehensively covered as part of a good foundation for future medical practitioners, it would be found deficient. But pain somehow is viewed and perceived differently, often in a discriminatory way.

Sometimes the knowledge and skillsets we utilize to test our trainees can be a good proxy for what we teach them. Designating pain as the 5th vital sign resulted in the need to teach those in clinical training about the importance of performing at least a cursory assessment for pain whenever we see a patient. What seems to have been ignored in many cases is teaching the best course of action is once the information about pain is obtained. The United States Medical Licensing Examination (USMLE) is a standardized examination that many states require for medical licensure. This examination is intended to assess knowledge and ability to apply that knowledge, and to determine proficiency in fundamental, patient-centered skills that are important in providing health care and disease treatment which constitute the basis of safe and effective patient care. One would imagine that with pain being as prevalent a medical condition as it is in the United States, that pain would be a prominent topic covered by this examination, especially considering the need for safe and effective treatment of pain. A 2018 analysis of pain and pain management-related content on the USMLE [4] examined question content related to pain. Of the limited number of examination questions which were related to pain, the majority focused on pain assessment and not on effective management strategies or the context of patients with pain. The authors point out that the challenge of reducing the burden of pain-related suffering and its intersection with the national overdose epidemic was paramount. Further, they reinforced that *"improved pain education for health care providers is an essential component of the multidimensional response to both still-unmet challenges."*

It seems as if there is something about pain that is not associated with the end of life or related to cancer that makes it "different" from the other medical conditions. This in turn can make clinicians think and act differently about it. It may be that pre-cognitively, we are somehow suspect of pain itself, the people who present with pain as their medical problem, or both. There may be many reasons why this is the case, but pain and its management just do not seem to fit into the paradigms and frameworks that clinicians often are taught to use to guide them for other common medical conditions. One reason for this could be because of the subjective nature of pain. In everyday clinical practice, the lack of measurable markers for the presence of pain (practical ones at least) means that we must rely on *the patient* to tell us how severe their pain is. We must **trust** the patient. We must **believe** the patient. We must consider that something we are forced to assess but cannot see is "**worthy**" of deeper assessment, diagnosis, and treatment. We must somehow incorporate this all into a planned course of action, with treatment recommendations that are derived through shared decision-making. We must be willing to tackle a medical problem that we may not have been adequately educated about.

One other important complicating factor in this dilemma is that in many cases, the scientific evidence necessary to form consensus and algorithmic treatment planning for pain is limited, controversial, or in some cases incongruent. Despite best intentions, 24 years have passed since 2000, when the affirmation of pain as a bona fide medical condition began with the promise of research to answer all the unanswered questions to come. Much of the controversy over these years has focused on the role of opioid analgesics in the management of chronic pain. The "**opioid pendulum**" has swung from one side to the other. Overdose fatalities have reached "epidemic" proportions, and position statements about when and how opioids should be considered as part of a pain treatment plan have vacillated and have been passionately debated, in many cases without scientific evidence basis.

Few would argue that pain *is* different from other medical conditions. There are several explanations for this, but this deviates from typical standard medical paradigms. If the context in which pain occurs affects how we approach it or *whether* we approach it, it may be that some recalibration is necessary. Unlike hypertension or hyperglycemia, if we are willing to assess and treat pain differently based on the person who is presenting with it, regardless of whatever their pain rating is on a scale of 0–10, then the care we are delivering may not be reproducible, equitable, and ethical. Maybe our past experiences, in some situations, tell us that the patient should just be able to "handle it", to "suck it up." Maybe it is because we don't believe the patient. Maybe it is because we collectively just don't know what to do because we didn't receive any education about it in our training. But it must be remembered that if we are at least coarsely assessing pain every time we ask the 0–10 question, and not addressing it, then the ethics of that decision-making process comes into question. If two patients have a similar pain-related complaint and we determine that one of them should be treated and the other not, then it should be a warning signal that somehow something may be wrong with our reasoning process and delivery of care.

Other aspects of pain make pain different. Pain is a self-reported symptom, sometimes clearly the result of an injury or associated disease process, and sometimes one that is unaccompanied by any evidence of any pathology or tissue damage. This sets the stage for the patient to have to somehow **prove** that their pain exists. This "burden of proof" can frequently be challenging for someone. Having pain severe enough to seek medical attention for it, and then having to somehow figure out how to get someone to believe that the complaint is valid can be difficult. With most other medical conditions, this burden does not exist. People with hypertension, heart disease, and other medical conditions are usually not in danger of being labeled a malingerer. If anything, in those situations, the patients are the ones who have to be willing to believe that something is wrong. Sometimes the end result is that patients may exaggerate their pain rating to reinforce just how much it hurts. It is not uncommon to ask a patient in severe pain what their pain rating is on a scale of 0–10 and have them reply "12″ to get the point across. This idea of needing to convince someone that pain is real is further confounded by the fact that in some cases, people may be fabricating their complaint of pain for some reason, whether it be medication-seeking, desire to not have to work, etc. Sometimes it can be for a clinician to know, especially in the absence of good foundational education about pain and its treatment. Skepticism about pain-related complaints sometimes abounds, and when it is coupled with stigmatizing thinking, behaviors, or beliefs and bias, the differences about pain become very apparent.

Another important contrasting aspect of pain compared to other medical conditions is that **the patient has a vote in the determination of success or failure of a treatment outcome**. This is a significant departure from "standard" common medical conditions and requires a mindset that is adjusted appropriately. It would seem comical to determine a high blood pressure, recommend some treatment for it, and then have the patient return for reassessment, find the blood pressure still elevated, and ask the patient for their opinion about how it should be managed. In fact, patients often rely on their healthcare professionals to make decisions about success or failure *for* them. Not so with pain. Once the patient is engaged in the assessment of the pain treatment outcome, navigation for the uneducated clinician can become even more challenging. Shared decision making and informed, nonpaternalistic care is the standard for medical care today. Unlike other medical conditions where the clinician's interpretation of information gathered generally dictates treatment planning and measurement of successful treatment outcomes for that patient, pain is not only something as clinicians we cannot objectively identify, but it is something that we also cannot make conclusions about regarding efficacy on our own. In fact, identifying mutually determined realistic goals and expectations of treatment is a critical component of pain assessment. If the clinician's goals and expectations do not align with those of the patient, the likelihood of successful treatment and satisfaction diminishes significantly. This deviates from most other medical conditions where clinicians explain the desired treatment outcome(s). This aspect of pain management may make many feel uncomfortable, and in some cases even frustrated with pain patients, leading us to want to avoid them altogether. And it needs to be remembered that this of course does not include the other pressures that impact pain and its treatment, like the overdose epidemic that is so prevalent in our country today, and intimately woven into the stigmas associated with pain and opioid analgesic therapy. This may be why these patients are often "the patient you least want to see." Considering that pain is so different from other medical conditions because it requires **belief, trust, patience, compassion, and affirmation**, sometimes in the absence of "proof."

Pain as a Disease

In 1953 John Bonica, one of the founders of modern pain medicine referred to pain as "a pathologic and destructive force that negatively impacts quality of life" [6]. Whether or not pain should be defined as a disease has been debated for years in medicine [8] In the context of acute pain, it may be reasonable to consider **pain to be a symptom** related to an injury, a nociceptive event (such as surgery), and a protective mechanism. If treated or given time to heal, symptomatic pain is often expected to likely resolve over time, along with other associated signs and symptoms such as swelling, redness, tenderness, etc. In this context, pain is considered to be adaptive, and it is reasonable that most clinicians and patients might not consider pain in these situations to be "a disease."

Merriam-Webster defines a disease [7] to be "a condition of the living animal or plant body or of one of its parts that impairs normal functioning and is typically manifested by distinguishing signs and symptoms." Regardless of its temporal nature (acute, subacute, or chronic), pain *may* impair normal functioning and *is* typically manifested by distinguishing signs and symptoms. It may then be reasonable to conclude that based on individual circumstances, at least in persistent situations, in the presence of some degree of neural and psychological reorganization, **pain *is* in fact a disease**. Numerous predisposing factors for the development of persistent pain have been identified and include genetic predisposition, central sensitization mechanisms, along with many others. In these situations, not considering pain to be a disease may potentially further the denial of people suffering with pain to be recognized as ill, and even their own ability to identify themselves as being ill.

The impact of pain from a societal and financial perspective is significant [9, 10]. More than 1 in 5 American adults experience chronic pain alone at any given time, and 1 in 10 American adults suffer from chronic pain which limits their ability to work to some degree, and significantly impacts their ability to perform normal activities of daily living. From an economic perspective, the estimated financial burden of lost productivity of chronic pain to society to be $296 billion each year alone, with the total annual financial burden estimated to be between $560 and $635 billion annually. Pain is the one of the most common reasons that Americans seek medical attention, and there are indications that this may continue to increase for a variety of reasons. Aging of the U.S. population likely will increase the prevalence and burden, as more people experience other common diseases with which chronic pain is often associated, such as arthritis, diabetes, cardiovascular disorders, cancer, etc. Greater public awareness about chronic pain syndromes may also increase the likelihood of someone seeking medical attention for untreated or undertreated pain.

Similar to other medical conditions, certain populations are at either increased risk for developing chronic pain or inadequate treatment for it. Increased vulnerability has been identified in people based on characteristics including level of health literacy, race, ethnicity, socioeconomic status, sex, gender, age, level of cognitive impairment, being a military veteran, etc. Social determinants of health, access to care, and other factors also can play a large role in adequate care.

Whether or not one considers pain to be a symptom, a disease, or both, it is a significant health issue in our country today, and for a variety of reasons has defied efforts to systematically define it, assess it, and in many cases, treat it.

References

1. The International Association for the Study of Pain. https://www.iasp-pain.org/. Accessed 16 June 2023.
2. Raja SN, Carr DB, Cohen M, Finnerup NB, Flor H, Gibson S, Keefe FJ, Mogil JS, Ringkamp M, Sluka KA, Song XJ, Stevens B, Sullivan MD, Tutelman PR, Ushida T, Vader K. The revised

International Association for the Study of Pain definition of pain: concepts, challenges, and compromises. Pain. 2020;161(9):1976–82.

3. The IASP Announces Revised Definition of Pain. https://www.iasp-pain.org/publications/iasp-news/iasp-announces-revised-definition-of-pain/. Accessed 16 June 2023.

4. Fishman SM, Carr DB, Hogans B, Cheatle M, Gallagher RM, Katzman J, Mackey S, Polomano R, Popescu A, Rathmell JP, Rosenquist RW, Tauben D, Beckett L, Li Y, Mongoven JM, Young HM. Scope and nature of pain- and analgesia-related content of the United States medical licensing examination (USMLE). Pain Med. 2018;19(3):449–59.

5. Chen JH. A PIECE OF MY MIND. The patient you least want to see. JAMA. 2016;315(16):1701–2.

6. Bonica JJ. The management of pain. Philadelphia: Lea and Febirger; 1953.

7. Disease Definition & Meaning – Merriam-Webster. https://www.merriam-webster.com/dictionary/disease. Accessed 16 June 2023.

8. Treede RD, Rief W, Barke A, Aziz Q, Bennett MI, Benoliel R, Cohen M, Evers S, Finnerup NB, First MB, Giamberardino MA, Kaasa S, Korwisi B, Kosek E, Lavand'homme P, Nicholas M, Perrot S, Scholz J, Schug S, Smith BH, Svensson P, Vlaeyen JWS, Wang SJ. Chronic pain as a symptom or a disease: the IASP classification of chronic pain for the international classification of diseases (ICD-11). Pain. 2019;160(1):19–27.

9. Institute of Medicine (US). Committee on advancing pain research, care, and education. Relieving pain in America: a blueprint for transforming prevention, care, education, and research. Washington, DC: National Academies Press; 2011. PMID: 22553896. ISBN 978-0-309-21484-1

10. Yong RJ, Mullins PM, Bhattacharyya N. Prevalence of chronic pain among adults in the United States. Pain. 2022;163(2):e328–32.

The Negotiation of Pain and Suffering

3

Advocacy and Pain Management

From an ethical perspective, there is virtually universal consensus that one of the key roles of a clinician (in addition to providing medical care) is to serve as an advocate for patients, their caregivers, and other family members. Sometimes, these actions of advocacy involve education, and other times they may altruistically involve expressions of compassion, empathy, and kindness. In all situations, and regardless of the patient's diagnosis, advocacy requires ethical recognition, fostering a sense of belief, trust, and respect. Applying these principles to pain and its management, with so much passionate discussion, debate, and controversy having transpired since 2000, it seems as if one consequence of the controversies surrounding today's pain management environment is that clinician advocacy for people with pain has either diminished significantly out of frustration or in some cases disappeared completely. This is despite the fact that an argument could be made that when caring for people with pain, the need for advocacy is even greater today than ever before. Unfortunately, for a variety of reasons discussed throughout this text, pain seems to be either ignored or minimized by many stakeholders today. But one important group of stakeholders that passionately continues to highlight the need for pain advocacy is people with pain. If we consider that pain affects patients not only biologically but also psychologically and socially, we must also be cognizant of the need for advocacy for all those inside the person-with-pain's immediate life and social circles.

Once the overdose epidemic started to impact regulatory and clinical pain management decision-making more significantly, the messaging about treating people with pain as a "moral imperative" of healthcare delivery began to change as well. What began with pain being designated the "5th vital sign" and a "Pain Patient Bill of Rights" to ensure appropriate treatment gradually transitioned towards messaging about the importance of a more restrictive approach to safe and appropriate prescribing of opioids and while still making sure to maintain access for those patients determined to be candidates for opioid analgesic therapy. Over time, this

© The Author(s), under exclusive license to Springer Nature Switzerland AG 2024
K. L. Zacharoff, P. Migdal, *Pain, Drugs, and Ethics*,
https://doi.org/10.1007/978-3-031-63018-7_3

transitioned to messaging designed to promote decreased opioid prescribing, de-prescribing or tapering opioid therapy, and negative messaging about long-term use of opioids altogether. The phrase "*while maintaining access to opioids for those patients in need*" was essentially excised from the landscape. It became clear that from a regulatory perspective, that decreased prescribing would undo the harms of liberal prescribing of opioids and lead to fewer overdoses and drug-related (or as some would say, opioid-related) fatalities. Messaging which has now shifted toward one goal—fewer opioid-related overdoses and overdose deaths.

Interestingly, the association between cancer-related pain and non-cancer-related pain has changed over time as well. Much of the work regarding pain treatment advocacy as is exists (or existed before) today can be attributed to the enthusiastic work of the American Cancer Society, and associated cancer-related advocacy organizations. With pain being such a frequent medical problem resulting from the cancer itself, cancer treatments, or both, building a sense of need for pain advocacy in this patient population was readily received. Cancer-related pain management was virtually universally considered to be an integral and necessary component of being able to deliver compassionate care to people stricken with the disease of cancer. Interestingly, nomenclature changed over time as well. Initially, terms like malignant and nonmalignant pain were used to differentiate between cancer and noncancer pain. Today, cancer and noncancer pain are the most commonly used terms to distinguish between the two. This increased level of pain advocacy spilled over to people with all types of pain, cancer-related or not. It seemed as if there was an ethical basis for providing pain relief to people with a disease like cancer, the same should also apply to the myriad of other types of conditions and diseases with associated pain. "Adequate pain treatment for all" was the mindset, with opioid analgesics to be utilized when necessary, and with a strong sense of advocacy for the somewhere between 60 and 100 million people stricken with pain. Cancer versus noncancer seemed to be less important of an influencer in clinical decision-making.

But as the paradigm of pain management (especially with respect to changing views about liberal utilization of opioid analgesic therapy) shifted, the delineation between the use of opioids for cancer and non-cancer-related pain shifted and, in some ways, re-emerged as well. Advocacy has stayed consistently strong for the unconditional safe and effective treatment of cancer-related pain with whatever means necessary. This may be due to the emotional biases that healthcare professionals and others have toward someone experiencing pain in the presence of the diagnosis of cancer, with few debating the ethics of providing opioids to patients with a diagnosis of cancer or taking whatever means necessary to provide adequate pain relief. More would increasingly debate what should be done for those with noncancer pain, and regulatory language once again started to refer to differences between cancer and non-cancer-related pain.

One of the best illustrations of this renewed delineation between cancer and non-cancer pain was the release of what most in the pain world refer to as "The CDC Guidelines" [1]. Titled *the CDC Guideline for Prescribing Opioids for Chronic Pain*, these were released in March of 2016 by the Centers for Disease Control and Prevention (CDC) and endorsed by the U.S. Department of Health and Human Services. These guidelines were intended for nonexpert (*not* pain specialists) clinicians considering treating patients with chronic pain with opioid analgesic therapy. Clearly stated in this document was the statement that the recommendations were intended for prescribing opioids for chronic pain "outside of active cancer, palliative, and end-of-life care." But even advocacy for patients with cancer-related pain may be diminishing as a result of the CDC Guidelines, with the adoption of them applying to all patients. A recently published analysis [2] of trends in opioid access among a large group of patients with poor prognosis cancer at the end-of-life revealed that opioid access had declined significantly between 2007 and 2017, with a corresponding increase of emergency department visits in this same patient population for treatment of pain during that time period. It may very well be that public policies designed to mitigate "opioid risk" in other patient populations is one reason for this troubling trend.

In any case, it would seem that we are at a crossroad with respect to advocacy for patients with pain, regardless of their diagnoses. As more people continue to succumb to drug-related overdose deaths, the desire from a public policy perspective may somehow be sacrificing the needs of patients with pain—cancer-related or not.

Suffering

Few would argue with Cassell's [3] assertion that "*the relief of suffering is considered to be one of the primary ends of medical treatment.*" What might be surprising is that not unlike pain and its management, medical education about suffering traditionally is under-represented as well. In fact, similar to the aforementioned inconsistencies that exist about the lack of congruency of how clinicians often define pain, it is unfortunately also common for there to be a lack of concordance about how suffering is defined as well. If one were to do an internet search for the word suffering, what would be found in many of the top search results is that **suffering is often defined in the context of pain**. In fact, it is fair to say that very often the majority of us think about pain and suffering together more often than we might think.

In his landmark paper *The Nature of Suffering and the Goals of Medicine*, Cassell asserts that it can sometimes be difficult for one to anticipate what a patient might describe as a source of suffering. But the patient needs to be asked that question in order to answer it. Despite the fact that even though clinicians might not often consider relief of suffering to be a realistic or expected primary pain treatment outcome, patients may often expect that it will. In fact, patients may not often distinguish between the physical and nonphysical causes of their suffering when seeking pain treatment as clinicians do, they just want "relief." The point is that even if clinicians have a difficult time entertaining the idea that suffering *is* an experience, as mentioned above, so must pain *be considered an experience*, and the possible treatment of pain and associated suffering should be identified in terms of magnitude, impact on the patient's life, and realistically and mutually identified goals and expectations. This means that there needs to be attention paid to perception of *both pain and suffering* to determine best courses of action address and distinguish the commonalities and differences between what is physically taking place and what the patient's mind is perceiving they are feeling. Patients *feel* **pain**, and patients *feel* **suffering**, and both are experiences that are more complex than just purely neurologic phenomena. Sometimes they correlate positively with each other (as one might expect), with increased pain leading to increased suffering. But in other cases, as Cassell points out, even though pain might be severe, suffering might be mild or even nonexistent. An example is the pain of childbirth, which although severe in rating, most often leads to a rewarding outcome, where suffering is low or absent. This illustrates well that what patients believe about their painful experiences can potentially impact how much they suffer as a result. Someone with moderate pain who is given a terminal cancer diagnosis may feel overwhelmed that things are out of control, and end up suffering much more than someone with severe pain.

Cassel asserts that a significant challenge in medicine is that as technology and patient needs impact the practice of medicine, and finding common ground between mind and body an important key to success. Indeed, if the **experience of suffering** is coupled with the **experience of pain**, it may be due to the fact that people may "feel" that their lives are not in their own control, that they are overwhelmed by their pain, or that their future life direction is uncertain. Importantly, Cassel also mentions two things that are critically important from a clinical perspective regarding the relationship between pain and suffering. First, **when clinicians do not validate the existence of the patient's pain, either because there is absence of objective findings to explain the pain, suffering may be more likely to occur** because the patient may start to distrust their perceptions. This is often the case when a psychological cause of pain is suggested. Second is that patients with chronic pain may often find over time that they can no longer discuss their distress with others because they fear that they may "start to sound like a broken record." Both of these instances can result in significant negative impact from a social perspective, leading to suffering in varying degrees of social isolation.

I have observed these situations related to pain and suffering often over the course of my career. In fact, I have often referred to one of *the biggest issues* facing people with nonacute pain (subacute or chronic) is **the fear of "not knowing."** When someone is injured acutely, it is common for many questions to race through their mind. How long will this pain take to get better? How long will it take before I can resume normal activity? What needs to be done to fix whatever needs to be fixed? etc. In these situations, the capacity for clinicians to address these common concerns is most often based on empirical predictions which are made by clinicians appropriately based on experiential observations of treatment approaches, average time needed to rest, heal, recuperate, etc. Alternatively, when pain is or becomes chronic, our capacity to predict the future may become less specific, and our ability to allay common fears about the future and well-being may be diminished or not possible at all. This can set the stage for fear to potentially magnify the degree of suffering that a patient experiences in the face of suffering related to their pain. If someone experiences pain due to an injury for example, and they have a low level of associated fear, they may be better able to confront the circumstances of functional limitations and recover. Alternatively, someone may experience pain and feel threatened and even catastrophize about its potential life-impact. This could lead to deepening fear, defensive motivation regarding physical activity, and feelings of their quality of life being threatened, which could lead to the perception of more severe pain along with mounting anxiety. This could then be followed by an increased level of arousal, preventive motivation regarding physical activity, and avoidance of physical and social activity leading to deconditioning, disability, depression, and increased suffering.

There seems to be a lack of clarity today in the clinical world about the intended "purpose" of pain management, often leading to miscommunication, misunderstanding, and overall dissatisfaction among patients *and* clinicians. It is common for clinicians and even researchers to promote the notion that "some degree" of improvement in pain rating is an appropriate goal. Arbitrarily, some have proposed that a 30% reduction in patient-reported pain rating is a reasonable proxy for successful pain control. The likely premise for this logic is rooted in the idea that the biomedical, reductionistic approach to managing acute pain will translate to a similar treatment planning and goals for pain rating in the subacute or chronic pain population and will be a reliable indication of a successful treatment outcome. What clinicians believe to be the case often transfers to what patients expect and remembering that patient assessment of successful treatment is important to consider. If patient goals are not met, then treatment is not likely to be considered to be successful by the patient. There are actually many situations where the reductionistic model of thinking about pain management does not apply, at least not by itself. Very often this may be the case because of suffering that accompanies subjectively-rated pain which often results from functional impairment, significant negative psychosocial impact, or some degree of both.

This means that pain assessment, reassessment, and mutually-identified pain treatment goals and expectations must consider functional and psychosocial impact, consider that improvement in suffering in this construct could potentially be equally or even more important than an improvement in pain rating.

The Negotiation of Pain and Suffering

For most clinicians, it is rare to think about a person with any specific type of pain, whether it is acute, subacute, or chronic without an expectation of some degree of accompanying suffering associated with that pain. In many ways, this relationship between pain and suffering is similar to that of suffering related to other medical conditions, and in other ways, it differs and is unique. From a clinical perspective, this unique relationship may require a change in thinking from traditional assess, treat, and re-assess strategies. This is not to infer that suffering associated with other medical conditions or diseases is any less important than suffering associated with pain, but it is important to consider that since pain is *both* a sensory and emotional experience that the relationship between pain and suffering may be unique and more nuanced. One contributor to this exclusive relationship might be that not only do people with pain feel the need to prove to others that their pain is real, but that they also often feel compelled to qualify and quantify the degree of suffering they are experiencing along with it. If pain is indeed to some degree a concept that people "learn" over the course of their lives, as stated in the IASP revised definition, it is also possible that people may "learn" the concept of suffering as well. Even though pain and suffering may often be used interchangeably, they are different things which require independent clinical attention, assessment, and sometimes treatment. Asking someone to rate their pain based on a scale of 0–10 does not take this intimate relationship into consideration, as most of us have likely seen at one time or another. If someone answers the question of how they would rate their pain on a scale of 0–10 with the answer "12", instead of reacting to that answer with in a judgmental or biased way, it might be worthwhile to consider that they are attempting to answer a different question. They may be trying to convey the degree of suffering that they are experiencing in the context of their pain and answering above the limit of the scale is one way to communicate that message. It is therefore worthwhile to consider that sometimes there is a need for people to convey the degree of suffering associated with their pain experience, and sometimes there is a need for people to convey the degree of pain associated with their suffering. If we consider that significant educational gaps exist in medical training with respect to pain, consider that educational deficits with respect to suffering in the context of pain exist as well.

A paper published in 2014 [4] focused on the relationship between pain and suffering and impacted my thinking and the way I instruct students and teach other clinicians about pain and suffering in a very significant way. Although the title may seem a bit complicated, *Cortical Plasticity Related to Chronic Pain in a Continuous Interaction of Neuronal and Mental Processes*, this article promotes simple ideas about the relationship between chronic pain and suffering in a relatively simple and meaningful clinical context. The author explores the intersection of the physiological, cognitive, and emotional aspects of pain, proposing that there is a basis for considering pain to be a **"neuro-mental" phenomenon** rooted both in the nervous system and the mind. The argument was made at the time this paper was published for a need for a new definition of chronic pain to reinforce and identify this relationship. Promoting the idea that *"nociception is not pain,"* and that *"sensation is not perception,"* this paper proposed that the experience of pain, or the "Pain Matrix" could be influenced significantly in a variety of ways by the external, dynamic network of a person's life consisting of things such as beliefs, culture, socioeconomic level, stress levels, etc. What resonated so deeply with me were not only the descriptions of the conceptual differences, but also the highly interactive and often fluid relationship between pain and suffering which need to be considered in clinical practice.

Although many might think that giving care to patients with pain requires a completely different clinical framework, advocacy and helping patients navigate the **negotiation between pain and suffering** is *not* dissimilar to the clinical paradigms for management and suffering associated with most other common acute or chronic medical conditions. There are often likely shared concepts, such as mutually identified and shared clinical goals, which involve helping the patient negotiate many hurdles including symptoms, challenges, lifestyle changes, and suffering that may be associated with any or all of them. Whether we think of diabetes, heart disease, or any other common medical condition, it is instinctive to want to do what Hippocrates is credited with suggesting: *"Cure sometimes, treat often, and comfort always."* Disruption in the patient's ability to continue to live pre-diagnosis has the potential to negatively impact patients' lives logistically, physically, and mentally. Helping patients manage goals and expectations is consistently a part of the delivery of informed, effective, and compassionate medical care. For some patients, adaptation will be easier, and for others it may be more difficult.

Helping patients navigate the negotiation of chronic (and even acute or subacute) pain and suffering means that we must broaden our assessment to allow ourselves to consider the impact that external factors, cognition, and emotions may have on the degree to which our treatment(s) is(are) focused. If we remember that the patient's mental and emotional states have the ability to impact the patient's perception of pain, it makes sense that it is possible that our assessment approach needs to capture information about those influencers in addition to the neurologic phenomena that are taking place. Sensation, perception, pain, and suffering can dynamically interact with each other in real-time and should all be included as part of a comprehensive pain assessment. Cultural background, past painful experiences, individual personality traits, beliefs, and economic conditions are all examples of external factors that can influence both sensation and perception. Someone's cognitive capacities, such as their ability to process information, pay attention, learn, reason, and make decisions are examples of cognitive factors that can also influence the relationship between pain and suffering.

From a clinical perspective, there are certain things that are unique and sometimes challenging in dealing with the negotiation of pain and suffering. Once again, this may be amplified due to the lack of comprehensive education that clinicians are exposed to during the course of their training. Most medical training programs (Physician, Nursing, PA, NP, etc.) prepare clinicians to consider the neurophysiological processes involved with pain. These teachings include focusing on the interaction between sensation, neuronal states, and perception—**the physical aspects of pain**. This prepares future clinicians for the implementation of treatment planning approaches similar to what would normally be utilized for other common medical conditions—assess, formulate, and recommend treatment based on a biomedical model approach.

Employing a "reductionistic" goal for pain treatment, this strategy emphasizes nociception as the main target and source of pain, and typically employs medical management in the form of pharmacologic treatment(s). While this may often be appropriate for many types of acute pain, little "negotiation" is involved. The metric of success is reducing the patient's self-reported pain rating (e.g., 0–10). Additionally, goals and expectations of treatment based on this model may often to some degree be paternalistic in nature—with clinicians recommending that the patient *"do what I say, and your pain will get better"*, and patients often asking, *"what should I do to help relieve my pain?"* or *"just tell me what to do so this pain can get better."* Often patient involvement is limited to reporting back in some prescribed period of time the degree of success, progress, or failure of the implemented pain treatment plan. In this situation, suffering, if present at all, is usually directly correlated with the immediate level of life-impact and degree of pain intensity, with "**the fear of not knowing**" not usually a cause or contributor to associated suffering.

While the aforementioned biomedical model may be often be satisfactory for patients with acute pain such as pain resulting from an injury or postsurgical pain, this model does not incorporate the intricacies related to the more complex negotiation of pain and suffering which may be involved in patients with subacute or chronic pain. What has been, and continues to be, problematic is that in the face of little to no education in medical training about how to approach persistent types of pain and suffering, clinicians may often rely on acute pain-relieving strategies when faced with assessing and treating patients with these persistent types of pain, which in turn may be inadequate and unsuccessful. Successful negotiation of pain and suffering in patients with subacute or chronic pain requires approaching assessment and treatment based on a **biopsychosocial model** as opposed to a purely **biomedical model**. This involves considering that central mechanisms are woven into the pain and suffering experience, requiring not only focusing on symptomatic complaints or pain ratings, but also on illness behavior and emotional responses to pain and associated suffering. Most often this will involve employment of a multidimensional, systems-based approach which, along with the utilization of pharmacologic agents and interventional approaches, will incorporate cognitive, behavioral, complementary, and self-management approaches. Self-management strategies can often be *critical* components of a persistent pain treatment plan, and passive clinician-directed treatments are rarely likely to achieve elevated levels of successful treatment outcomes or patient satisfaction. Failure of the patient to engage in self-management strategies as part of the treatment can often be a sign of a low level of motivation, which in many cases predict a lower likelihood of successful treatment and patient *and* clinician satisfaction, having a negative impact on the relationship, communication, trust, and capacity for advocacy.

Pain, Suffering, and Quality of Life

A discussion about pain and suffering would not be complete if it did not also include the impact of pain and suffering on overall quality of life (QOL) (See Fig. 3.1). QOL can differ significantly from one patient to another, which is why context is such an important part of a comprehensive pain assessment. Certainly, from a purely

Fig. 3.1 Pain, Suffering, and Quality of Life

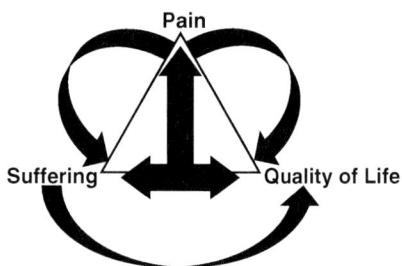

epidemiologic and socioeconomic perspective, pain and suffering have the potential to significantly impact QOL to some degree for all patients, but the individuality of patients based on their life context, including activities of daily living, and goals and expectations related to pain management outcomes can vary tremendously. For some reason though, a byproduct of traditional healthcare educational curricula, or pain-related deficits in healthcare education, many healthcare professionals consider pain and the "pain experience" to be different from the traditional "illness experience" associated with other common physical and medical problems. This mindset also has the potential to result in differing clinical impressions about the impact of pain on QOL versus those resulting from other common medical conditions.

General consensus is that training has prepared clinicians to expect that when patients experience an illness or a physical problem, or they are informed about a serious diagnosis, that there will be a resulting cascade of mental processes that go through the patient's mind along with their own associated adverse effects. These processes include **initial awareness of a diagnosis or a physical problem**, often followed by some degree of **distress**, which then may result in some type of **"illness-related behavior,"** with the patient taking **on the role of being "sick."** These are all expected processes that a trained clinician is taught to expect and help the patient deal with, or in some cases even to confront. These concepts are not complex and are universal. But when patients present with a pain-related complaint or diagnosis, even though it should be expected by the healthcare professional that a similar behavioral cascade will occur, it may not, and that has the potential to negatively impact patient care. This is despite the fact that in 1989, Loeser and Egan brought the similarities and relationships to light [5]. They discussed in detail the relationship between **nociceptive events**, **the experience of pain**, **ensuing degrees of suffering**, and **pain-related behavioral processes** which parallel those observed with traditional illness behaviors. This should not have been groundbreaking, even back in 1989, but it was. Unfortunately, while this was shared with clinicians in the pain community, like many other aspects of pain education, it was not widely shared or taught to most frontline practitioners. The end result may have contributed to a frequent lack of clinical consensus about pain and its impact on QOL.

Given the fact that someone's assessment of their pain may be subjective, assumptions about the associated degree of suffering and overall impact on QOL might be inaccurate if other information is not gathered as part of the patient assessment. There is a growing, but slowly-disseminated, consensus that pain affects the person as a whole. QOL is defined as the person's evaluation of their well-being and **physical and emotional functional capacity**. This is exactly the reason pain management outcomes should not be measured purely in terms of reduction in pain ratings. Additionally, it should not be assumed that pain is synonymous with decreased QOL. Alternatively, it can be assumed that pain can have significant adverse effects on QOL [6]. Aspects of QOL which are most commonly affected by pain include the logistical availability of health and social care, mobility, ability to work and/or perform activities of daily living, negative mood, disorder of sleep patterns, dependence on medication or other therapeutics, and sense of physical safety and/or security. It is important to consider that pain affects important aspects of the patient's perception of well-being and functionality. The most important word in the prior sentence is "perception." Perception of life-impact is the key, and individual to each and every patient. Additionally, it becomes evident that it will likely rarely be sufficient to solely treat only the pain rating, and that mitigation of suffering and increase in QOL will require directly targeting all areas negatively impacted. Equally important to pain-related QOL may be helping the patient identify areas of their lives *not* directly impacted or changed by their pain, such as spirituality, religious beliefs, etc.

Given the fact that chronic pain commonly occurs in the presence of other medical conditions, it is important to consider that comorbid conditions may significantly impact the degree to which pain impacts QOL as well. Depending on the specific comorbid disease or medical condition, pain might be expected or unexpected, and that in and of itself can have influence on QOL; "expected pain" may temper the impact pain has on QOL, because the element of surprise or The "fear of not knowing" can be potentially mitigated to a certain degree. Alternatively, "unexpected pain" may have a more negative impact on QOL. Additionally, depending on the medical condition (e.g., cancer-related pain), pain or increased pain may often be perceived as advancement of disease, and regardless of the pain rating, may negatively impact QOL.

The same construct can be applied to pain treatments, outcomes, and QOL. Successfully approaching goals and expectations of pain treatment modalities are likely to postively impact perceptions of treatment effect on QOL, whether the patient's pain rating is reduced or not. Treatments which potentially negatively influence the aspects of QOL (most importantly functionality) may have paradoxical effects on perception of QOL.

Individual patient differences can impact the relationship between pain, suffering, and QOL as well. These differences include age, cultural background, socioeconomic status, learned pain behaviors, and coping skills to name a few. Depending on the circumstances and despite pain rating, functional capacity and social dynamics may be affected significantly or not at all given the exact same pathophysiologic and other variables. Once again, this fortifies the rationale for gathering this kind of information as part of a comprehensive pain assessment. It is important to remember that beyond the effect that pain can have on physical activity and function, perceived impact that pain has on QOL may also be measured by effect on emotional state, social capacity, and cognitive functioning as well. It is important to consider that helping a patient to successfully navigate the intimate relationship between pain, suffering, and impact on QOL my involve approaches which minimize these effect that pain has on these domains of life, once again justifying a concerted, multidisciplinary, medical, *and* biopsychosocial approach to effective pain management.

References

1. Dowell D, Haegerich TM, Chou R. CDC guideline for prescribing opioids for chronic pain—United States, 2016. MMWR Recomm Rep. 2016;65(RR-1):1–49.

2. Enzinger AC, Ghosh K, Keating NL, Cutler DM, Landrum MB, Wright AA. US trends in opioid access among patients with poor prognosis cancer near the end-of-life. J Clin Oncol. 2021;39(26):2948–58.
3. Cassel EJ. The nature of suffering and the goals of medicine. N Engl J Med. 1982;306(11):639–45.
4. Fernández-Salazar M. Cortical plasticity related to chronic pain in a continuous interaction of neuronal and mental processes. 2014.
5. Loeser JD, Egan KJ. History and organization of the university of Washington multidisciplinary pain center. In: Loeser JD, Egan KJ, editors. Managing the chronic pain patient. New York: Raven Press; 1989. p. 3–20.
6. Niv D, Kreitler S. Pain and quality of life. Pain Pract. 2001;1:150–61.

Biomedical and Biopsychosocial Approaches to Pain and Its Management

4

Background

As mentioned earlier in this text, many healthcare professional training programs do not specifically devote a significant amount of training to students that is devoted to pain and its management beyond a simple pain assessment rating (e.g., NRS 0-10). This could exist for a variety of reasons, but is somewhat counterintuitive given that pain remains one of the most common reasons that people seek medical attention in the United States today. One would think that given the prevalence of pain that it would be part of the core curriculum of training programs. From a clinical perspective, often clinicians in practice or clinicians in-training often express exasperation about having to pay "more attention" to pain because there are so many other things that typically need to be addressed as part of a comprehensive primary care or front-line practitioner patient visit, and there is just not enough time to justify an appropriate amount of attention to anything beyond capturing the cursory pain rating. I think that some of the conflict in many people's minds is that back when pain was designated the 5th vital sign, it was implemented without the buy-in from clinicians, who in many cases were lacking appropriate education about pain and its management. The end result was that this information (the pain rating) was often captured without much foundational knowledge about what to clinically "do" with it. I have had many clinicians tell me that their training was most often geared toward the competency examinations they would have to take to assess knowledge and clinical skills. As mentioned in Chap. 2, an analysis of the USMLE as an example showed that most questions on the examination focused on the assessment of pain, and not much more beyond that.

This sets the stage for clinicians to apply existing paradigms which are typically utilized in the assessment and treatment of other common medical conditions to pain and its management. In simpler terms, this is an overlay of a model which approximates the mindset of assess, test, diagnose, formulate treatment plan, implement treatment plan, and then reassess. In most cases, both clinicians and patients likely expect the treatment plan to include something which could *not* be obtained in the absence of the clinical interaction—a prescription for something; usually a medication. Certainly,

© The Author(s), under exclusive license to Springer Nature Switzerland AG 2024
K. L. Zacharoff, P. Migdal, *Pain, Drugs, and Ethics*,
https://doi.org/10.1007/978-3-031-63018-7_4

this prescription could be for some kind of physical or behavioral therapeutic component of treatment, but in most cases this prescriptive treatment will involve the employment of some type of pharmaceutical component to help treat the "chief complaint" or associated symptom(s), sign(s), and/or diagnostic findings related to the diagnosis of the medical condition. In many cases, in fact, patients to some degree consider the prescription of a medication to be the "reward" worth the effort involved with making the office visit and going through the effort of having the clinical interaction take place. In essence, in many cases, our healthcare system in some ways is designed to have pharmaceutically based or **biomedical approaches** to healthcare be foundational parts of both patient and clinician expectations. An important question to consider is whether this model translates effectively to the treatment of pain.

The Biomedical Approach to Pain Treatment

There is a high likelihood that prior to patients seeking medical attention for most nonserious or life-threatening pain-related complaints, a variety of self-treatment strategies have already been employed by the patient which will often involve taking some type of medication, most commonly those available over the counter without a prescription. People are essentially putting into practice a biomedical approach to self-management of pain. These medications commonly include nonsteroidal anti-inflammatory drugs (e.g., aspirin, ibuprofen, or naproxen), acetaminophen, or a variety of other over-the-counter pharmaceutical options. Alternatively, there is a subset of patients who may wish to avoid taking medications at all costs, and will likely self-direct available nonpharmacological or physical approaches, such as heat, ice, massage, exercise, etc. Either way, it is reasonable to think that in many situations, the biomedical paradigm of reducing pain as a purely nociceptive event with pharmacologic and nonpharmacologic therapeutics is somewhat "baked" into the mental processes of people who are managing their pain even *before the first clinical visit*. This mindset is then often reinforced by the prescription-based biomedical reductionistic approaches which clinicians will employ when patients present to their clinical setting.

There are two main points to consider in a bit more depth. First, that the biomedical model for managing pain traditionally approaches pain whether acute (1 month duration or less), subacute (more than 1 month but less than 3 months), or chronic (3 months or longer) as a purely nociceptive phenomenon, even though this model is likely only appropriate for the treatment of acute pain. This "mechanistic" strategy typically focuses on physical and or neurological mechanisms, applying a "reductionistic" approach using diminished subjective pain ratings as the sole metric of successful treatment outcome. Second, that the biomedical model typically builds a treatment plan that is founded upon medical (pharmacologic) management. Clinicians and patients alike consider these both to be the de facto way to assess and treat pain. If unsuccessful initially, generally alternative pharmacologic treatments may then be substituted, and the medication-based cycle continues. If we consider that mutually-defined (clinician and patient) goals and expectations of pain treatment are critically important in the context of pain treatment outcomes, then it may be fair to say that clinicians who have received little to no education about pain and its treatment may collaboratively suggest and affirm patient expectations about the principal role of pharmacologic treatments and reducing pain ratings as a metric of success for all types of pain, regardless of its etiology, location, or duration.

By nature, clinicians often tend to employ treatments and strategies most familiar to them, which have worked in the past for other patients, and that they have come to clinically trust. Almost reflexive in nature, the thought processes and algorithms used for other ailments and medical conditions often result in clinical recommendations that are streamlined, intuitive, quick, and from a thought-process perspective, less disruptive. The biomedical approach to pain treatment is familiar to most clinicians and patients because *it is* just that—familiar. This construct conforms to conceptual models which harmonize with knowledge and prior clinical experience. It is therefore not surprising that to clinicians using a biomedical model that it is "comforting" because it applies to so many other common medical situations and does not seem out of ordinary practices. Furthermore, if we consider that this approach is what patients often expect to take place, something that deviates from this path may seem disruptive to them as well. Criticisms of the use of the biomedical model to treat all types of pain and patients are numerous. They include that mistakenly focusing on being reductionistic with respect to subjective pain ratings and solely relying on tissue damage and nociception as frameworks is an approach that is oversimplified, unsophisticated, not individualized, and that it may potentially result in marginalization of patients with no identifiable pathophysiologic cause of pain (idiopathic pain).

The fact that the biomedical approach to pain treatment has limited value in all but the most acute types of pain underscores why education of healthcare professionals is so important to efficacious pain management. Additionally, the role of healthcare professionals as patient educators is critical in helping patients to calibrate realistic goals and expectations that are rooted in much more than just a biomedical approach to treating pain—more than a simple medication prescription.

The Biopsychosocial Approach to Pain Treatment

In 1980, Dr. George Engel published an article about the clinical application of the biopsychosocial model in medicine [1]. Dr. Engel referred to biomedical approaches being ingrained in the fabric of medical education and that they are to a certain degree "taken for granted" and assimilated into clinical practice framework for all medical conditions. Exploring the relationship between clinician and patient, this article identifies that relationship as a complementary one, with roles of a party in need (the patient) and a party with the ability to provide an expected set of responses or services (the clinician). In this "mechanistic" interaction, expectations are that the clinician's knowledge of science and available diagnostics will provide necessary answers and solutions to meet the patient's needs.

Regardless of the level of clinical sophistication, few would likely argue against this rationale because in many situations this approach realizes desired outcomes.

Proponents of an illness experience-based, biomedical approach to virtually all common ailments claim that when researchers provide enough information there will be refinements in the mechanistic interaction, with patient-tailored treatment planning increasing the reliability of treatment outcomes. Critics of the mechanistic approach argue that entirely basing assessment, diagnosis, and, most importantly, treatment planning may ignore what can be the single most unifying quality of all patients with any medical condition—the humanity of the patient.

In the area of pain and its management, in the past many have argued that if clinicians were able to "drill down" to the pathophysiologic root of pain, tailored treatments would be more successful. In most cases, this refers to neurological, physical, and/or chemically mediated aspects of pain, and treatment planning is based on mitigating one or more of them. When the year 2000 was designated as the beginning of the *Decade of Pain Control and Research*, it was *precisely this premise* that was the impetus for this declaration, for research to provide the unanswered questions about pain mechanisms.

What seems to have been ignored are the other important pieces of information that patients (and sometimes clinicians) bring with them to the clinical interaction in addition to their medical concerns and pathophysiological anomalies—the context of their lives in the presence of the pain-related complaint(s). These are the individualized components of the assessment that help to **understand the patient** in pain, **instead of *understanding the pain*** in the patient, with the latter assuming that the pain in the patient is somehow isolated from the circumstances surrounding the person with pain. In fact, so many variables exist in the context of the patient with pain, that it is likely that rarely if ever would two patients with the same pathophysiology or pain complaint ever be exactly alike in terms of their contexts. It follows that the formulation of an individualized treatment plan would also not likely be the same. If pain is truly both a nociceptive *and* an emotional experience, then an attempt to categorize patients with pain algorithmically would infer that emotionally and neurologically they are "identical," which is highly unlikely or virtually impossible to be the case. It is worthy to note that this applies to any type of pain, whether it be acute, subacute, or chronic.

An uncomplicated way to think about this is within the framework of mutually- (patient and clinician) determined pain treatment goals and expectations. If several patients with the same or similar identifiable pathophysiology and pain-related complaint present to a clinic setting for treatment and evaluation, it might be the case that the clinic or healthcare system's desire is that they be "plugged-in" to pain care paths, clinical algorithms, etc. This disregards the differences that might exist, such as cultural differences, socio-economic status, age, gender, health literacy level, employment status, occupation, and religious and spiritual beliefs, to name just a few. A purely biomedical approach does not consider medical comorbidities, psychological comorbidities, the patient's level of motivation, genetic variations, stressors, or other potential clinical influencers. Certainly, this might make sense from an efficiency perspective, but if you consider the number of permutations, the likelihood that someone's goals and expectations of pain treatment could be the same as someone else's is quite low. For example, the goals and expectations of pain treatment of a recently retired 70-year-old executive could be to be able to play a round of golf every day, to travel to visit their grandchildren, or just relax on the sofa. Alternatively, if another patient with the exact same pain-related problem and symptom profile presents who is a 39-year-old mother who is a stay-at-home care-taker of three young children, it is highly likely that the goals and expectations of pain treatment may be significantly different based on life circumstances and age alone. Add to that a history of anxiety, catastrophizing behavior, depression, rela-tionship problems, or other life stressors, and it is not hard to imagine the variation that could exist in their desired pain treatment outcomes. Sometimes the differences may be more subtle. Two similarly aged high school students with the same knee injury and resulting pain could have quite different concerns and desired outcomes based on their responsibilities (such as work) or extracurricular activities (such as sports). If this patient-specific information is not captured or considered to be rele-vant to the assessment process, then it might result in ultimate miscalibration of treatment planning and desired outcomes.

Biopsychosocial approaches to treating pain must include much more consider-ation than just information gathering about pain and context of activities of daily living. A patient's unique social background can significantly impact treatment decisions, patient desires, and patient goals. This includes things such as a person's cultural background, social environment, economic factors, and the presence or absence of a healthy social support system.

For a clinician to apply the biopsychosocial approach to pain management to clinical practice, it is important to consider that the relationship with the patient is critical. In fact, in most cases, the quality of this relationship can help determine the ability to identify level of motivation, self-awareness, and expected level of adher-ence to a pain treatment plan. It is also imperative to consider that self-awareness could be valuable not only as a diagnostic, but also as a therapeutic tool. And when taking a history, it is always important to elicit information in the context of the patient's life circumstances.

The spectrum of psychosocial context of pain is broad. A biopsychosocial model focuses on central mechanisms instead of peripheral/nociceptive ones. Illness behav-iors, including cognitive impact and emotional responses to pain are important con-siderations. Once this information is gathered, decisions can be made based on the dynamics of the biological, psychological, and social domains that are particularly valuable in promoting the patient's pain management, incorporating a multidimen-sional, multi- *and* interdisciplinary plan of pain treatment. Consider things like **bio-graphic disruption** of the patient's life with a **reconstruction of their narrative**, and some adjustment in their living that has ocurred due to their illness that is pain.

Something that may often be overlooked in taking a pain-focused history is the patient's capacity and willingness to participate in self-management strategies to manage their subacute and chronic pain. To a certain extent, acute pain management is to a certain degree paternalistic by nature, in that *passive* participation is required of the patient—if the patient follows directions, their pain will likely improve. Subacute and chronic pain treatment plans which are founded on biopsychosocial pain management require *active* patient participation, specifically with respect to self-management. There is an much lower likelihood of successful pain treatment without patient participation.

Consider that managing pain is really a negotiation of the pain itself, the degree of suffering experienced by the patient, and an intimate interaction of the patient's bio-psycho-social dynamic. This may often be further complicated by factors such as regulatory scrutiny, stigmatization, and issues that by design may hinder adherence to a pain treatment plan.

The Pain Escape Plan

Most agree that pain most commonly serves as a protective mechanism, acting as an alert to identifiable and immediate threats. Pain protects by quickly allowing for actions that prevent further harm. From that perspective, it can be thought of as a neurologic "alarm system." When a painful stimulus occurs, it is **transduced** into a signal that can be **transmitted** to the spinal cord, where there may or may not be some degree of **modulation** (dampening or enhancement) of the signal, and then ultimately **perception** of pain at the cerebral level, which then promotes defensive behavior. Alternatively, fear is commonly considered to be a protective emotional reaction to an identifiable and immediate threat as well, protecting an individual from harm by promoting defensive behavior(s). Fear is comprised of **interpretation** of something that is threatening, **sympathetic arousal** (e.g., "fight or flight" phenomenon), and produces **defensive behavior(s)**.

When these protective mechanisms are working "normally," they act in concert to protect us from harm. When one or both become abnormal, they may work together to promote avoidance behaviors that end up losing their protective nature, potentially leading to undesired outcomes.

This is another illustration of the intimate relationship between the biological, psychological, and social dynamics, and how the combination of pain and fear and may lead to what is sometimes referred to as the "**reflexive experiential pain escape plan**" [2]. When a person is injured and pain is an accompanying symptom, it is likely that virtually everyone will have some type of pain-related "experience." When a painful experience occurs, many people may suffer not only because of the pain itself and associated physical impact, but they may also suffer because in many cases, there may be a "fear of not knowing" how long the experience will last, what their limitations will be, and how long they will last, and whether there will be long-term consequences or not. It is reflexive to think about how long someone might be "out of commission" or the things they will and will not be able to do until they recover.

From that point on, it is possible that a patient will experience a relatively low level of fear associated with the pain and accompanying behavior changes, confront them, and, from both a physical and psychological perspective, recover. What is important to keep in mind is that fear is an individual response, and not due to any specific aspects of the injury or nociceptive phenomena taking place.

Alternatively, following a pain-related experience, it is possible that some degree of expected fear may transition to an "abnormal" state of catastrophic thinking, called **catastrophizing**, which is the process where anxious patients dwell on the most extreme consequences possible. It is possible that this catastrophic behavior may be triggered by receiving news about the injury or pain that is perceived as threatening, but it is also possible that the person's life circumstances may serve as the fuel. Catastrophizing may then lead to an increased fearful thinking including an **increased level of arousal**, **perception of threat** (to normal living), and **"defensive" motivation** (such as becoming negatively motivated to participate in the pain treatment plan or physical rehabilitation, etc.). This sequence may then lead to **increased perception of pain**, development of **anxiety**, or both, which will include an even **higher level of arousal**, **hypervigilance** to prevent pain, and a shift to "**preventive" motivation** (such as avoiding activities, social interactions, etc., in an effort to prevent increased pain and/or disability). These behaviors may lead to increased measures to avoidance behavior, diminished activity, and decreased level social interactions and "escape," which may then lead to physical **deconditioning**, **increased disability**, and in some cases, **depression**.

Which path a patient follows after the pain experience may not be completely controllable, but it is important to consider things from a clinical perspective which might be influential. It is important to consider the need to identify certain behavioral characteristics that make a patient more likely to experience deviation from the "normal" path, with the intention of preventing these fear-avoidance behaviors before they occur. There may also be predispositions or "vulnerabilities" which may tilt the balance toward one path or the other that should be identified as part of the assessment process. They may include: **genetic predispositions**, which can impact and exaggerate the behavioral expression or physiologic responses to pain; **generalized biological vulnerabilities**, which may lead to increased stress, cortisol release, and decreased modulation of serotonin and/or norepinephrine; **generalized psychological vulnerabilities** such as the presence of anxiety or personality disorders, which may impact the ability to accept living with pain, adherence to treatment plans, and lead to increased suffering and decreased motivation; or **social vulnerabilities** such as being under- or uninsured, lacking means of transportation, or experiencing stigmatization resulting from prejudice(s). These may potentiate the perception and sensation of pain in a variety of diverse ways including increased allostatic load or enhanced peripheral and/or central sensitization. Once again, this means that digging deeper than just the standard pain-related history for these traits and incorporating components into the treatment plan that consider them is no less important than identifying the nociceptive-based treatment plan components.

It is also possible that fear-avoidance behaviors may be inadvertently fueled by the interaction between patient and health care professional during a clinic visit or other communications. This could result from subtle body language (such as facial expressions to answers to certain questions or findings in the history and physical), or the use of certain diagnostic terms which could be fear-inducing due to their level of complexity or perception of seriousness by the patient. It is also possible that there could potentially be transference of fear-avoidance thinking from the clinician either based on their own past personal or clinical experiences. This underscores the importance that clinicians need to reflect on their own beliefs and biases, not only to provide equitable care and offer all possible treatment options, but also to avoid the negative psychological consequences of fear-avoidance behaviors that could potentially result.

In summary, to a considerable extent pain *and* fear are most often protective, adaptive mechanisms. If one, the other, or both somehow become dysfunctional and lose their protective nature, they may significantly and negatively impact pain treatment outcomes. It is incumbent to gather information that is much more detailed than pain intensity, location, and duration. It should be considered similar to how important it is to identify other comorbid medical conditions. There may be concurrent fears and concerns that a patient has which could have tremendous importance on a patient's quality of life. These include stressors resulting from diminished functional capacity, inability to work, financial concerns, and decreased ability and/or desire to engage in social interactions.

This illustrates the importance of employing a multifaceted biomedical and biopsychosocial approach to managing pain in a multidisciplinary and interdisciplinary manner when possible. As mentioned previously, it is important to keep in mind that when it comes to pain and its management, the patient has a powerful voice in dictating what is a successful or unsuccessful treatment outcome. This fortifies the importance of considering a patient's psychosocial context in addition to the physical one, not only in the pain assessment process, but also in the development of a pain treatment plan and its likely ultimate trajectory.

References

1. Engel GL. The clinical application of the biopsychosocial model. Am J Psychiatry. 1980;137(5):535–44.
2. Leeuw M, Goossens ME, Linton SJ, Crombez G, Boersma K, Vlaeyen JW. The fear-avoidance model of musculoskeletal pain: current state of scientific evidence. J Behav Med. 2007;30(1):77–94.

Roles and Responsibilities of Stakeholders

5

Background

Over the past 20 years, many strategies to improve the quality and safety of pain treatment have been explored by several "key stakeholders." Sometimes these strategies had a variety of competing and sometimes even conflicting methodologies and intentions, including promoting the most judicious safe and efficacious use of opioid analgesics, increasing the employment of nonpharmacologic pain treatment modalities when appropriate, helping to better achieve optimal pain treatment outcomes, and not least importantly helping to mitigate the increasing wave of overdose deaths plaguing the United States today. During this same period of time, there has also been a significant amount of finger-pointing and controversy among appointed and, in some cases, self-appointed "stakeholders" who gained a significant amount of momentum once pain was designated the 5th vital sign. The result of "muscle-flexing" and input from these "stakeholders" has had a significant impact on clinical practices and patient care over these two decades.

In some ways, identifying stakeholders, especially the most important ones, has become quite a complex process and even sometimes a confusing exercise, even though one might think it seems simple to identify who the appropriate stakeholders are or should be. Indeed, if a stakeholder is defined as a person or group with a special or invested interest or concern, it is not hard to imagine that there are many who have laid claim as "stakeholders" in the complicated world of pain management and substance use. If recognizing stakeholders can be somewhat difficult, it stands to reason that establishing roles and responsibilities of involved stakeholders can become more complicated as well. One could easily imagine that with the number of stakeholders increasing significantly over the years, similar to other situations in life, the more groups "seated at the table," the harder it may be for them to reach consensus.

This chapter will identify and give some brief examples of "key" stakeholders, and their roles and responsibilities, but should in no way be interpreted to be comprehensive—they are too numerous to count. However, *it is important to underscore that one group* of stakeholders is and has always been an unchanging constant, one

© The Author(s), under exclusive license to Springer Nature Switzerland AG 2024
K. L. Zacharoff, P. Migdal, *Pain, Drugs, and Ethics*,
https://doi.org/10.1007/978-3-031-63018-7_5

group whose voices should rise above all others in terms of key significance—*people* with pain. While this may seem to be self-evident, common sense, and not necessary to mention, it is important to remember that many times, as hard as it can be to imagine, people with pain are often completely left out of the equation as stakeholders. Yet, if every discussion, debate, regulatory decision, guideline, recommendation, etc., does not consider the patient with pain to be *the most important* **part of the equation**, then the mission and purpose of those activities can lose their ethical focus and, in many cases, lose sight of their moral directives as well. Sadly, it is *not* uncommon (*and even likely in many cases*) for this unintentional exclusion to occur in the current environment of pain, substance use, and the overdose crisis. Understandably, passions and tensions related to leaving people with pain out of the discussion often tend to run high. In fact, what happens in many cases is that patients with pain often feel abandoned, and are often subjected to stigmatization, ridicule, bias, and labeling, which frequently leads to poor levels of communication, socialization, productivity, and isolation and worsened suffering.

It is not uncommon for professional meetings consisting of those who are most often considered to be "key stakeholders" to be convened without patient inclusion and representation in the educational discussions, deliberations, and decision-making processes, even though they are potentially the ones most likely to be affected by the outcomes. For example, frequently, when guidelines or practice recommendations are deliberated, created, and released that pertain to the management of pain, prescribing of opioids, or employment of other treatment options, groups of experts in the field are brought together to develop them and create consensus around them. Rarely, if ever, is consideration given to how information about these recommendations or their rationale will ultimately find its way to direct patient care with an adequate level of communication and understanding. Instead, the focus is usually centered on transmitting this information to clinicians about new "standards of care," many times with a major emphasis on potential liability in the absence of adherence to new recommendations, guidelines, or imposed regulatory requirements and standards. In most cases, the job of passing this information along to patients falls on the shoulders of clinicians who are often (appropriately) fixated on avoiding things like regulatory scrutiny and experiencing frustration (in many cases) resulting from the constraints being placed upon them. Instead of educating patients about the rationale for circumstances and changes in practice, clinicians often just dictate the "rules" to patients.

In some situations, there have been instances where the effects of "knee-jerk" reactions to regulatory stakeholder mandates along with educational deficits at the clinician level have had chilling effects on the management of pain. One such example is when the federal government looked to the Center for Disease Control and Prevention (CDC) for help in mitigating what was then referred to as the "opioid epidemic," which was presumed by the government to be the result of indiscriminate or liberal prescribing of opioids to manage pain. The result was what are now referred to by many as the "CDC Guidelines," which were developed by the CDC to guide opioid prescribing in a primary care setting for the treatment of chronic noncancer pain which, were published in 2016 [1]. The overarching messages from these "guidelines," as they are often referred to, found their way to clinicians through a variety of different regulatory stakeholder channels, in an inconsistent and often confusing fashion. In some cases, this was through scientific literature, and in others it was through the mainstream media. In some cases, with little or no modification at all, certain state medical boards adopted and incorporated these "guidelines" verbatim into their practice standards for opioid prescribing in their state, with the result being that if clinicians didn't adhere to them, there could be any range of potential repercussions resulting from admonishment or an investigation by the State Medical Board, the Drug Enforcement Administration, or both. Some of the most important messages of the CDC Guidelines were interpreted to be that diminished prescribing of opioids, tapering opioids prescribed chronically, and ceilings for morphine milligram equivalents (MMEs) in a primary care setting were critical to help mitigate the ever-increasing rise of drug-related fatalities in our country, many of those involving an opioid. Where things went awry in this example were the lack of roles and responsibilities of dissemination of this information to those who should have been considered as the most important stakeholders, *the patients*. People with acute and chronic pain who were being managed in primary care settings on chronic opioid analgesic therapy were often informed only at the time of refill request that their current dosing regimens were going to be abruptly decreased, tapered, or even in some cases discontinued due to "new guidelines." Reasons given to patients in many instances were that this was mandated by "regulators," who were perceived to be the most important stakeholder because authority had the capacity to put clinicians "on notice." The intentions were unquestionably good— there indeed was a well-documented relationship between increased prescribing of opioid medications after pain was designated the 5th vital sign and increasing numbers of overdose deaths in the United States. Even though causality was sometimes heavily debated, the correlation between the two seemed clear. This will be discussed in more detail in other chapters of this book, but it serves as an illustration of how patients were somehow left out of the creation of these guidelines and state mandates, even though they ethically should have been considered as *the most important stakeholders*.

One other point that is important to make is that if the hierarchy of stakeholders can sometimes be unclear or confusing, and it stands to reason that roles and responsibilities of stakeholders may then often be unclear as well. This chapter will attempt to discuss some of the most identified stakeholders and illustrate their roles and responsibilities as such.

Patients as Stakeholders

It seems logical to think that in the framework of roles and responsibilities of pain and its management, the *only* two important stakeholders should be *patients and the healthcare professionals* involved in their pain care. As mentioned previously, one of the unique characteristics of pain and its management is the fact that unlike other medical conditions, patients have a significant role in determining whether the treatment is a success or a failure. If every treatment option is crafted toward successful pain treatment outcomes, then patients are ***the most important stakeholders***, and their goals and expectations of pain treatment should take priority over everything else. From an ethical perspective, this also makes sense. As will be discussed subsequently in another chapter, all patients with decision-making capacity have the right to make autonomous choices about their medical care, and what their desires are with respect to pain treatment.

Unfortunately, in the real world of pain management, the equation is often not so simple. Very often, patient goals and expectations about pain treatment outcomes may differ significantly from those of the treating clinician. This situation could exist for a variety of reasons, with many other factors influencing clinician practices today. Additionally, as mentioned earlier, patients or patient representatives are not often well represented at regulatory meetings or education-related discussions about the development of public policies, clinical practice recommendations, or guide-lines, making underrepresentation a problem as well. The result often contributes to patients feeling that there is a need to "prove" that their pain symptoms are real, credible, and worthy of medical attention. People with pain usually completely understand the subjective nature of pain, and that objective findings alone do not solely support making a diagnosis. This makes one of the patient's responsibili-ties to be to figure out how to best balance expressing their complaints with an additional responsibility to convey their goals and expectations for treatment, along with conveying impact on overall quality of life. From a clinical perspective, this can sometimes be more challenging than it may seem, because very often patients only answer the questions asked of them, especially when clinician time and resources are taxed. If clinicians do not inquire about more than just a patient's pain rating on a scale of 0–10, then it is likely that the stage is not set for other informa-tion to be captured, and that does not necessarily respect the patient as a stakeholder as well. In many cases, patients might answer the question about pain rating on a scale of 0–10 with "12", hoping that it will convey the severity of the pain-related symptoms. Reactively, clinicians may then judge patients, label them as complain-ers or exaggerators, or precognitively make conclusions that portend a low likeli-hood of successful treatment.

In their roles as stakeholders, whether educated or not, patients ultimately have **two main responsibilities** when being treated medically. The first is **advocacy;** patients must be willing to advocate for themselves persistently, effectively, rationally, and, if possible, vocally. Unfortunately, as with many things, this may sometimes be easier said than done, especially when the person is suffering from pain which is severe. Even in the best-case scenario, regardless of the medical condition, advocacy can be a challenging task. It would seem that the single biggest advocate patients have should be their clinician, but if clinicians are worried about their own professional liability or other responsibilities related to clinical practice (i.e., opioid prescribing), it is possible that their capacity for patient advocacy may be deflected entirely or significantly diminished. The second most important responsibility patients have is a high-level of **adherence and participation** in their treatment planning and implementation. Patients have a responsibility to demonstrate the understanding of, and their ability to adhere to, a treatment plan that is mutually developed with their treating clinician, and to raise questions or concerns when they exist. This is quite different than following orders that are directed to them in a paternalistic way. In many cases, this responsibility requires patience, motivation, and a high desire for effective levels of communication and trust in the clinical relationship. If there is a situation where the patient is not able to adequately live up to these responsibilities, they may fall on the shoulders of caregivers if available, but they nevertheless remain the same.

It is also important to consider that patients may not often be aware of the differences in expertise or regulatory restrictions of primary care practitioners treating pain compared to specialists, and often may feel frustrated by delays in diagnosis, refusals to prescribe, or referrals to specialists for treatment with extended wait times for an appointment. The resulting dynamic often created may be one where patients feel that they are not often given advice or information, but instead given "rules" about what can or cannot be done, and informed of punitive measures that will be taken if those "rules" are not followed. For example, if patients see a sign in a medical office waiting room or are asked to sign a document stating that "opioids will not be prescribed here," they often may not understand the reason(s) for it, how best to response to it, and in many cases may appropriately end up feeling overwhelmingly negatively about it. Another consideration is that patients may not often understand the clinical reasoning behind urine drug screening as part of a safe and effective pain management treatment plan with opioid analgesics or other prescription pain medications. They may likely conclude that urine screens are being utilized as "lie detectors" to catch them. With the myriad of recommendations and guidelines, such as those recommending that prescribers check the prescription drug monitoring program database when prescribing controlled substances, it is more than likely that patients may often have no idea that prescription drug monitoring programs are used in all 50 states as safety mechanisms, or comprehend the reasons are for their use, other than to identify someone who might be getting multiple prescriptions from multiple healthcare providers.

A patient's understanding of their roles and responsibilities as stakeholders often come from trusting and privileged discussions with their treating clinicians about these and the many other principal issues that managing pain, substance use, and addiction present to clinicians and patients today, in a manner that facilitates understanding the rationale behind every measure taken. A request for a urine sample should not invoke different feelings in patients based on the clinical circumstances, whether it be in the context of an annual physical examination, or in response to a request for a prescription refill to ensure safety and effectiveness of opioid therapy. If patients perceive possible punitive complications, they may be more likely to react to it as such. This can often be counterproductive and lead to a diminished sense of trust, transparency, and ultimately clinical success. It often falls on the shoulders of clinicians to help patients understand the clinical rationale, to help make them effective stakeholders, and to be cognizant of their roles and responsibilities as key stakeholders.

Clinicians as Stakeholders

Our healthcare system is built on the premise that what takes place in the context of a clinical encounter between a patient (and/or their caregiver) and their healthcare provider is privileged and that ideally from an ethical perspective provides the patient with a decision-making process which is autonomous, informed, comprehended, and mutually-derived based on a trusting relationship which facilitates understanding of risks and benefits, patient consent, and awareness of roles and responsibilities of all parties involved.

A significant amount of attention has been paid by healthcare over the last two decades to promote the paradigm that patient care is delivered with the intention of assuring the patient that they have a "medical home" which will provide them with a medical sanctuary. Pain care is no different from other types of medical care in this regard. Not surprisingly, most of the care for people with pain is provided by frontline, primary care clinicians who are perfectly positioned to provide patients with the same sense of comfort and security. With approximately 60 million people in the United States with chronic pain [2] and approximately 5000–6000 Board Certified Pain Specialists in the country, simple math dictates that there is often no other option for patients than to seek pain treatment from their primary care clinicians. In fact, even in situations where a patient is experiencing postsurgical acute or subacute pain, primary care clinicians are often looked to be the center of pain treatment in the absence of abnormal recovery, postoperative complications, delays in healing, etc.

In the absence of comprehensive education and training about pain and its treatment, this can sometimes be taxing for those primary care clinicians. There are other challenges clinicians face as well. Ideally, medical decisions are made with complete transparency between a clinician and the patient, with risks and benefits to the patient ethically guiding that process. Patient risk and benefits are the guiding principles for autonomous decision-making. For a variety of reasons, as stated elsewhere in this text, when it comes to the management of pain, there are many other issues that exert forces on this risk/benefit analysis beyond just patient-level risks. For example, the prevalence of substance use involving prescribed opioid analgesics, and the increasing numbers of drug-related overdoses and overdose fatalities have increased the scope of risks and benefits far beyond those of the patient alone. Today as key stakeholders, when clinicians decide that a patient with pain may be a candidate for a trial of opioid analgesic therapy, it is incumbent on the clinician to consider that the scope of risks and benefits extends much further than just the patient, *especially* the associated risks. Clinicians must consider risks related to introducing the opioid into the household, and whether members of the household may potentially be at increased risk of an aberrant drug-related behavior, accidental ingestion, etc. Clinicians also must consider the risk that they may incur from the perspective of regulatory scrutiny.

The roles and responsibilities of clinicians involved in pain care have been quite dynamic over the past 30+ years. In the late 1990s, it was not uncommon for clinicians to be successfully sued for failing to treat or undertreating a patient's pain. In many cases, especially in the absence of an educational foundation, clinicians responded by liberally prescribing opioids to better meet the needs of patients with pain, and to protect themselves from litigation. The term "opioid pendulum" was coined to describe a period during which discriminating prescribing of opioid analgesics shifted to liberal prescribing of them, and then ultimately, in the face of the increasing "opioid crisis," shifting back to more discriminating prescribing practices, or in some cases, choosing not prescribing them at all—a "swinging pendulum" of opioid prescribing of sorts [3]. Basically, healthcare professionals who have chosen to provide pain care for patients have had to ride the "swing" along with other external pressures placed on them.

Gourlay and Heit published what is still considered to be a groundbreaking article which proposed using a "Universal Precautions" approach to providing pain treatment to patients with chronic pain in 2005 [4]. If these "precautions" had been widely disseminated or incorporated into educational training curricula back when they were published, it is very possible that the trajectory of pain management might have been different. Their recommendations did an excellent job of considering external forces clinicians face when treating people with pain and detailed how to implement a standardized approach to roles and responsibilities for clinicians treating pain. They were:

- To make a **diagnosis** with an appropriate differential
- To perform a **cursory psychological assessment** to determine the appropriateness of incorporating a biopsychosocial approach to treatment
- To **assess risk** of development of aberrant drug-related behaviors
- To obtain **informed consent** by facilitating understanding of risks and benefits of courses of treatment
- To either verbally or in written form clearly delineate roles and **responsibilities** of all parties involved
- To include a pre- and post-treatment plan **assessment** of pain rating and **functional capacity**
- To conscientiously **consider the role of opioid analgesics** as a component of therapy with or without adjunctive treatment approaches
- To **reassess** pain and function along the continuum of treatment
- To regularly **assess** analgesic efficacy, activity levels, presence of adverse effects, and presence of aberrant behaviors
- To consider that **pain and its pathophysiology are dynamic** and may change over time, along with the development of comorbid conditions, including addictive disorders
- **Documentation** of all the above to fulfill regulatory requirements and potential liabilities

It is important to note that these roles and responsibilities do not represent a significant paradigm shift for healthcare professionals because they are not dissimilar to those employed for other medical conditions, and therefore should not seem unsettling to most. Importantly, they provide a framework that applies to all patients regardless of pharmacologic deployment, have the potential to reduce stigma by treating all patients in a similar fashion, and can contribute to what many consider to be the most important task of all, minimizing overall risk.

Advocacy Groups and Membership Organizations as Stakeholders

Advocacy groups have frequently been a critically important voice and source of support for people suffering from a particular health-related problem. The range of services these groups provide varies but often proves to be invaluable for people and caregivers who just do not know where to turn to seek information and/or assistance. In some cases, advocacy groups direct patients toward verified disease-related educational resources and materials, and in others they may act as a lobbying voice to policymakers on behalf of the people they represent.

When it comes to pain and drug use, advocacy groups have often been particularly vocal and passionate about communicating the specific needs or challenges to policymakers and representatives of healthcare systems. One example of a large pain patient advocacy group has been the American Cancer Society (ACS). Even though its primary mission is devoted to battling cancer and its treatment, the ACS has played an important role in pain management. As mentioned previously (one of the many recurring themes in this text), pain was designated the 5th vital sign in 2000 in response to several different circumstances. At that time, there was a valid concern that many patients with cancer-related pain were often undertreated or untreated for their pain, regardless of whether the pain was related to the pathology, the cancer treatment, or possibly both. With a significant and impactful lobbying effort, the ACS became a voice for helping to shed light on existing pain treatment deficiencies and increased understanding among policymakers and regulators about how vitally important successful and compassionate pain control was to a cancer patient's overall quality of life [5]. One of the leaders of this lobbying effort was June L. Dahl, PhD. Dr. Dahl was a professor of Pharmacology at the University of Wisconsin Medical School, in Madison Wisconsin, and firmly believed that pain control needed to be, and *could* be better. She played a pivotal role in developing the Wisconsin Initiative for Improving Cancer Pain Management, a voluntary effort which was one of the first of its kind, if not *the first* of many State Pain Initiatives which are devoted to improving the quality of pain management for patients. The message promoted by Dahl and the Wisconsin Initiative was that while many effective pain-relieving medications were available for patients with cancer-related pain, they were either underutilized or given infrequently for reasons that included lack of clinician education about how to assess and manage pain, fear of addiction, and/or a lack of focus on pain and awareness about palliative care. Many consider Dr. Dahl to be instrumental in having the World Health Organization designate the Wisconsin Pain Initiative as a demonstration site which could serve as a model for improving the treatment of cancer pain in the United States and around the world.

Dr. Dahl and her colleagues' work was successful in lobbying for improved pain care in cancer patients in the late 1980s and early 1990s, and is often credited with becoming the cornerstone for identifying the need for pain control in the noncancer pain patient population as well, which ultimately culminated in pain being given its "vital sign" status. Despite the debate about whether this designation ultimately was beneficial or not, this example underscores how much impact an advocacy group can have on policy development and clinical practice. Speculation continues to exist today about how different things might have turned out if the call for attention to be paid to pain and substance use education had been as successful back then. Many claim that the 5th vital sign designation was created as either a marketing strategy by pharmaceutical companies to get clinicians to prescribe more opioid analgesics, or by the Joint Commission on Accreditation of Hospital Organizations (JCAHO), but those claims are purely speculative at best. The overdose epidemic seems to have obscured the sequence of events leading Congress and the Veteran's Health Administration to make that designation, and just how vital a role advocates for improved pain treatment in cancer patients played as stakeholders in making it happen.

Clinician membership organizations also have had a significant role as stakeholders, with significant impact on how pain and substance use is viewed and treated both in the United States and around the world. Examples include the International Association for the Study of Pain (IASP), The American Academy of Pain Medicine (AAPM), and the American Medical Association (AMA) to name a few. In some cases, criticisms have been made related to funding received from pharmaceutical companies for pain-related educational activities, and the effectiveness of some of these organizations as stakeholders has been limited or in some cases caused the organization to fail completely. One example of a stakeholder "failure" is the American Pain Society (APS). With its relatively large multidisciplinary membership, the APS was the U.S. national chapter of the IASP. In 2009, picking up where Dr. Dahl and her colleagues left off in their mission to promote better control of pain in cancer patients, the then highly regarded APS published a joint set of clinical guidelines with the AAPM for the use of chronic opioid therapy in patients with noncancer pain [6], with the intention of providing evidence-based recommendations underscoring the importance of clinical skills and knowledge in the safe and effective prescribing of opioids and the risks associated with drug use, addiction, and diversion of controlled substances. These guidelines were the product of the analysis of a multidisciplinary panel of 21 experts who were screened for potential conflict of interest, with the project being "entirely funded by the APS." The guidelines were rational, in that they (much like Gourlay and Heit's Universal Precautions recommendations) provided a reproducible set of steps that could be followed in clinical practice to mitigate the effects of educational deficits of most practicing clinicians at the time. These were heralded and referred to very positively for the next few years by most, especially since they were jointly created by what were then the two largest pain-related clinician membership organizations in the United States—significant stakeholders.

Unfortunately, the increasing number of lawsuits related to the "opioid crisis," criticism about liberal opioid prescribing practices, and questionable marketing strategies by pharmaceutical manufacturers of opioids, eventually enveloped the APS [7, 8]. Many lawsuits named the APS as a co-defendant for its role in helping to "fuel the fire" of the overdose crisis by promoting "liberal prescribing of opioids" along with the discovery that a significant portion of its revenue was from financial support from opioid manufacturers, which critics deemed as a direct conflict or potential conflict of interest, which then led to questioning of the underlying intentions the 2009 APS/ AAPM opioid guidelines. In 2019, the APS President at the time, William Maixner, DDS, PhD announced that the APS would cease operations despite the fact that it "promoted multidisciplinary research and clinical care in pain diagnosis and management since 1978" due to its "resources being diverted to paying staff to comply with subpoenas and other requests for information and for payment of legal fees instead of funding research grants, sponsoring pain education programs, and public policy advocacy." Many in the pain community felt this to be somewhat ironic as the APS was considered by many to be a stakeholder well positioned to help navigate the scientific evidence gaps, along with fostering research that could and improve pain treatment, prevention, and risk of substance use. The Academy of Integrative Pain Medicine (formerly known as the American Academy of Pain Management) suffered a similar fate for similar reasons, ceasing its operations in early 2019 as well.

The important take-home point is that advocacy groups and membership organizations have in the past and continue today to play an important role as stakeholders in the environment of pain, drugs, and substance use.

Regulators and Policymakers as Stakeholders

Regulators and policymakers have played a large role in how pain is assessed and treated, how prescription pain medications are prescribed, how substance use, substance use disorders and addiction are assessed and treated, and also in how tactics and strategies are deployed to stem the tide of increasing number of drug-related overdose deaths in the United States. It is important to define the composition of this particular group of stakeholders, as it may be more diverse than one might initially consider. It is also important to consider that sometimes the issues are much more complex and intertwined than one might think as well. For example, a case in point would be managing pain at the end of life, and how medications are used in that context.

Regardless of the definition or the intended purpose, policymakers have had and continue to have a significant impact on clinical practice and patients with pain and substance use. Many consider an important starting point in the role of policymakers to be 1971, when the federal government passed and implemented a law titled **The Federal Comprehensive Drug Abuse Prevention and Control Act of 1970 (also known as the Controlled Substances Act or CSA) [9].**

This law consisted of three main "titles":

- **Title I** which dealt with the establishment of rehabilitation programs for "drug abusers"
- **Title II** which addressed the registration and distribution of controlled substances
- **Title III** which addressed issues related to the import and export of controlled substances

The goals of the CSA were to improve the manufacturing, distribution, and dispensing of controlled substances and to be enforced by the **U.S. Drug Enforcement Administration (DEA)**, with input from the **U.S. Department of Health and Human Services (HHS)**. The CSA created five different "drug schedules" or categories: I, II, III, IV, and V. Any interested party was also given the opportunity to petition for a scheduling change, including pharmaceutical manufacturers, medical or pharmacy membership organizations, advocacy groups, state or local government agencies, and even individual citizens. These schedules were based on consideredation of the following factors:

- Actual or relative potential for unhealthy use
- Scientific evidence basis for a drug's pharmacologic effect
- The state of current knowledge regarding the drug
- A drug's existing history and current pattern of unhealthy use
- The scope, duration, and significance of unhealthy use
- Associated public health risks
- Liability of psychological or physiological dependence
- Whether an immediate precursor of the substance was already controlled in a scheduled category

Basically, the CSA mandated the DEA to become a significant stakeholder to make rules, regulations, and decisions about regulating and enforcing how clinicians prescribed controlled substances, and how prescription and illicit drug use could and should be dealt with. Over the years, the DEA has played a substantial role in this regard in pain management, most notably involving opioid analgesics and how they are used in the context of treating acute, subacute, and chronic pain, along with their potential role in substance use disorders, addiction, and the overdose crisis.

The **U.S. Food and Drug Administration (FDA)** plays a role as a key regulator policymaker stakeholder, with a federal mandate for its mission to be to protect public health. The difference between the FDA's role as compared to the DEA is that most of the influence of the FDA is typically directed toward the manufacturers of medications, such as opioid analgesics for pain treatment, substance use, and addiction treatments. In this regard, the FDA has served as the counterpart to the DEA in terms of evaluating safety and efficacy of prescription medications and plays a role in assessing the potential for unhealthy use and addiction when that potential exists. Additionally, when considering controlled substances for approval, the FDA includes a determination and recommendation for drug scheduling to the DEA.

In recent years, there has been some crossover with respect to FDA policies and its role directly impacting clinical practice and patient care, particularly evident with respect to the prescription of opioid analgesics [10]. The FDA's role does not conclude with pre-approval and approval; it actually extends over the entire life of the drug, and in the case of substances that are deemed to have a higher liability for unhealthy use, the FDA has the responsibility to implement and oversee strategies that it mandates to mitigate this risk, including clinical educational activities. Originally, this was most commonly in the form of requiring drug manufacturers to present a detailed "**risk management plan**" as part of the drug approval process. This evolved into the FDA requiring a more comprehensive approach to mitigating risk of unhealthy use, addiction, and overdose related to long-acting/extended-release opioids called **Risk Evaluation and Mitigation Strategies or REMS**. The REMS included a "blueprint" for clinician education about these formulations of opioids and was comprehensive in its curricular scope. FDA required that the funding for development and dissemination of these educational activities was to be provided collectively by the manufacturers of these products, with specific success metrics from the FDA along with outlining a detailed timeline for the creation and implementation of these activities. One major challenge with this approach was that the FDA did not have the authority to mandate that all prescribing clinicians must participate in these educational activities. That authority typically rests with the DEA. Another challenge was that many felt at the time that opioid REMS education should cover the use of *all* opioids, including short-acting/immediate release formulations. Lastly, grants were provided to individual organizations to develop and disseminate their own versions of the REMS education, which while based on the FDA's blueprint as a core requirement, offered differed substantially content in some cases. In many cases, clinicians who did participate in one REMS education program were confused, uninformed, or both about whether they should engage in another activity with a different name, which one they should choose, and the potential for redundancy. Even though the FDA ultimately made the decision years later to have the REMS include education and activities devoted to safe prescribing of all opioid formulations, many still question the successfulness of this approach in mitigating opioid risk.

Other federal stakeholders worthy of mention include the **White House Office of National Drug Control Policy (ONDCP),** the **Substance Abuse and Mental Health Services Administration (SAMHSA),** and the **National Institute on Drug Abuse (NIDA).**

The ONDCP creates policies, priorities, and objectives for the nation's drug control program, with the intention of reducing illicit manufacturing and use, diversion, and drug-related crime and violence. Working closely with the DEA and FDA, through its **National Drug Control Strategy**, guidelines are created and implemented to facilitate cooperation among federal, state, and local authorities to address and prevent substance use through education, substance use treatment delivery, and enforcement.

SAMHSA, part of the U.S. Department of Health and Human Services, is the lead federal agency for addressing issues related to substance use and mental health. In addition to providing educational materials and resources, SAMHSA is also responsible for providing primary source information to other agencies about the incidence and prevalence of substance use in the United States.

NIDA is the lead federal agency supporting scientific research on drug use and its consequences, with its core mission being to advance science on the causes and consequences of drug use and addiction and to apply that knowledge to improve individual and public health through a variety of mechanisms, including disseminating of information and education.

At the state level, a key stakeholder is the **Federation of State Medical Boards (FSMB)**, an organization that supports the individual state medical boards in licensing, disciplining, and regulating physicians and other healthcare professionals with the intention of "keeping patients safe." Recognizing inconsistencies in pain care and opioid prescribing across different states, the FSMB developed its own **Guidelines for the Chronic Use of Opioid Analgesics** [11] to provide a uniform set of recommendations that would help clinicians "understand the relevant pharmacologic and clinical issues related to the use of opioid analgesics," including how they should be safely prescribed, the role of other multimodal treatments, and the importance of states providing sufficient, targeted continuing education to achieve these goals.

Payers as Stakeholders

Employing several different strategies to control cost and minimize risk including formulary restrictions, need for prior authorizations, quantity limits, and co-pays, payers can exert significant force as stakeholders in pain management and substance use treatment. In many cases, payers are not included in discussions about guidelines, recommendations, or even education, which many times creates the opportunity for significant confusion and frustration about the intersection of best practices, insurance coverage, and reimbursement.

The Pharmaceutical Industry as Stakeholders

The manufacturers of medications used to treat pain and substance use disorders are stakeholders by virtue of their liability and responsibility as dictated by many of the stakeholder groups mentioned above. Many of the actions taken by the stakeholders above directly impact almost every aspect of the pharmaceutical industry, whether it is by complying with compulsory practices which proactively promote public safety or regulations specific to drug scheduling. Coupled with the increasing overdose crisis our nation faces, opioid manufacturers are challenged now more than ever to ensure that risk mitigation efforts and stewardship are more comprehensive than ever before, while still trying to innovate, conduct research, and development. Not excluded from this equation are responsibilities to create initiatives which promote education and increased awareness among clinicians, patients, and caregivers about public health concerns related to abuse, addiction, etc. Additionally, ongoing surveillance about these issues with reporting data to the FDA and DEA are responsibilities of these stakeholders as well.

Educators as Stakeholders

It is reasonable to think that when most people think about relevant stakeholders involved in issues surrounding pain treatment, substance use, and even ethics in pain care, educators are not often considered significant or considered at all. Yet, lack of education and foundational knowledge in any disease state or medical condition is one, if not *the* most important barriers to optimal assessment and treatment. In fact, after patients, **educators may be one of** the *most important* **stakeholders** of all, if one subscribes to the mindset that education is the foundation upon which all of these and desired outcomes rest. Education may be one of the only durable successful strategies that can be taken to address so many of the issues which have persisted with respect to pain and drugs over the past 20 years. It is widely known that medical disciplines place a significant level of importance on education throughout the course of a clinical career. Continuing education is routinely required virtually across the country to maintain licensure, medical privileges, etc. Given the prevalence and burden of pain, the skyrocketing number of cases of substance use, overdose fatalities, and concerns about addiction and its treatment our healthcare system and society face today, it seems somewhat contradictory that **foundational education** about these and related topics are frequently not given the attention they deserve in the training of future physicians and other healthcare professionals today. If pain is one of the single most common reasons that people seek medical attention for, how could it be possible, for example, that medical students could complete their undergraduate training with little or no education about pain, its management, substance use, and addiction?

As mentioned in Chapter I, Mezei et al. published findings about the quantity and consistency of pain and substance use education in medical schools across North America in 2011 [12]. Thirteen years later, not much has changed with respect to that, despite many regulatory efforts over these same 13 years designed to educate clinicians already in practice. Voluntary educational activities about these subjects have not been successful in attracting participants or changing practice behaviors for a variety of common-sense reasons. Lack of sufficient time and resources are the most likely culprits for this lack of success, but confusion is sometimes the reason as well. In typical fashion, many different stakeholders (e.g., the FDA, the DEA, and SAMHSA) have created a variety of educational programs that sometimes are consistent and other times inconsistent in their educational missions and messaging, with the result being that instead of being complementary to each other, in some cases they have been *competitive* with each other. Instead of logically building an educational program that is longitudinal, they have been "one and done" activities that do not necessarily achieve a meaningful and enduring educational goal. Many states across the country have now made some portion of required continuing education about pain or opioids a requisite for license renewal, but again without specific goals or direction, and more in a "check the box" way without much consideration to changing practices or improving care.

If we consider that multidisciplinary management of chronic pain using a blended biomedical and biopsychosocial model has been shown to be better positioned to achieve desired outcomes *and* more cost-effective [13], it seems contradictory that they are not more commonly employed or more widely available. Reviews of the literature about stakeholder's opinions about this have reported a variety of reasons to explain this, including utilization of resources, economics, etc. Most importantly though is that most stakeholder groups believe that clinicians often lack the training they need to achieve these goals. Additionally, these groups reported that this lack of education has resulted in many *patients* believing that healthcare professionals often lack the relevant knowledge to provide optimal pain care, and that the educational deficits have led to general practitioners to consider that pain is not a disease in its own right, and that its management is less of a priority than other medical conditions, and that pain patients will often be nonadherent to treatment plans more often than other patient populations.

It is important to note that the need for education of future healthcare professionals in the areas of pain management, substance use, and addiction has been publicly endorsed widely since 2000, with 2011 being an example when the White House Office of National Drug Control Policy (ONDCP) released its report titled *National Drug Control Safety* [14] which underscored the importance of education about pain and substance use in clinical education to mitigate the nation's drug crisis. Virtually *any* set of practice guidelines or recommendations related the management of pain, opioid prescribing, and substance use treatment released within the past 15 years reiterates that many of the challenges we face today could be at least partially addressed by making pain, substance use, and addiction part of the compulsory core curriculum in health profession training programs.

A more recent example emphasizing the importance of educators as key stakeholders is the 2019 report titled ***Pain Management Best Practices*** published by the Pain Management Best Practices Inter-Agency Task Force [2], convened jointly by the U.S. Department of Health and Human Services, the U.S. Department of Defense, the U.S. Department of Veterans Affairs, and the ONDCP. This report stressed that more effective education and training about pain and its treatment is critical, and should occur at *all* levels of clinician training, including undergraduate training (e.g., medical school training), graduate professional training (e.g., internship and residency training), and continuing professional education. Additionally, this report underscored that the utilization of all types of pain treatment approaches, including medication-based treatment, restorative therapies, interventional procedures, behavioral therapies, and even complementary and integrative health approaches were ultimately informed by the implementation and effectiveness of clinician training.

Clinicians have responsibilities as educators for their patients as well. Despite the wealth of information available via the internet, patients still rely mostly on their healthcare professionals to provide them with the information and education they need. For clinicians to be effective educators, it makes sense that they need to have received education on these topics themselves. This is not meant to refer to expert-level pain specialists or addictionologists who are likely to be well-trained and well-informed, but to frontline general practitioners, on whose shoulders most of this burden as educators often falls. Additionally, for clinicians to build a trusting relationship with patients that includes open, honest, and effective communication, a good clinical educational foundation is key, especially when topics like pain and substance use are so widely covered by the mainstream media and may create so many questions and controversies in people's minds.

From an ethical perspective, the process of informed consent cannot occur in the absence of education and effective communication. When treating pain, often early diagnosis and intervention is crucial, but lack of adequate training may lead to acute pain which may not be optimally treated, increasing the likelihood of progression to subacute or chronic pain which, in turn, may also be inadequately diagnosed and managed. This may lead to several negative consequences, not the least of all increased suffering, and in many cases chronically debilitating conditions. Educational deficits in pain medicine have other effects as well including the lack of a standardized pain assessment and significant barriers to patient-provider shared decision-making and treatment planning.

The roles and responsibilities of educators at the intersection of pain, drugs, and ethics is critical. This education needs to be standardized, well-structured, and considered to be analogous to the use of seatbelts when teaching someone to drive an automobile. This education needs to take place in the formative years of clinical training, and across the variety of disciplines that make up the patient care team, including physicians, physician assistants, nurse practitioners, nurses, therapists, psychologists, pharmacists, and many others. People often only consider the relationship between the physician and the pain patient when it comes to health education, but nothing could be further from the truth. Today, for example, pharmacists are considered to play an ever-increasingly vital role in education, and safe and effective delivery of pain care. Additionally, in many cases, caregivers need to be involved in the educational process as well, as in many cases, their level of education may be vitally important.

Naloxone and its use when opioid analgesics are prescribed underscores the importance of the roles and responsibilities of education in pain care. Naloxone has been widely recommended for consideration to help address one of the most serious adverse events associated with opioids, respiratory depression. In fact, in December 2018, after a 2-day meeting, the conclusion and recommendations by the Anesthetic and Analgesic Drug Products Advisory Committee to the Food and Drug Administration resulted in the Department of Health and Human Services issuing a guidance [15] to all prescribers that naloxone should be co-prescribed to patients at higher risk for an opioid overdose, and discussed with other patients for whom opioids are prescribed, with concomitant documentation of the discussion, rationale, and conclusion about whether to co-prescribe naloxone or not. From the perspective of education as stakeholders, there are several points to be made. Primarily, that many clinicians were in many cases not aware of this guidance at all. There was no consistent, uniform mechanism for dissemination of this information in the form of educational materials to clinicians in practice, or future clinicians in training about this guidance and its recommendations. Further, there was little, or no attention, paid to how patients and caregivers could or should be instructed about how to use naloxone, or how to identify someone who was an appropriate candidate for its use. Just the fact that naloxone is unlikely to be used by the person for whom it is co-prescribed means that education of others who might be the ones to administer it is a critical piece of the puzzle, and certainly a factor that could potentially influence the effectiveness of naloxone in helping to prevent adverse events, and even death. The presence of naloxone in the household is not going to save lives, but knowing how, when, and why to use it could make all the difference, even down to the idea that naloxone is intended to be a bridge to emergency care, and *not* as an antidote, which mainstream media often implies.

This is just one example of how the effectiveness of education flowing from clinicians to patients and caregivers could be substantially impacted by lack of education to the clinician.

Another illustration of how educators and education play a leading role in pain management, substance use disorders, and addiction is related to storage and disposal of opioid analgesic medications. Virtually all regulatory agencies recommend that when opioids are prescribed that patients are to be instructed about **storing them in a safe place**, out of reach of other individuals, who might suffer harm from them, or use them in an unhealthy way, for example to get "high." Additionally, **it is against the law for anyone to share a controlled substance** that is prescribed to them with *anybody* for any reason. Education about this needs to come from the prescriber, but education about the importance of conveying this information as part of the informed consent process is often lacking. Think about whether you or one of the members of your household has ever been prescribed a prescription pain medication, and whether this educational information was provided or not. With respect to disposal of controlled substances, such as opioids, the same applies—it is the duty of the prescriber to be educated about proper disposal, and when the medication should be disposed of. Again, consider whether you have received or witnessed education about this topic as well.

Telling someone to wear a seatbelt in a car because it is the law is not the same thing as letting them know *why* it is important. We live in a world today where words matter more than ever before, yet from a perspective of terminology, and incorrect use of words, likely from a lack of education, inaccurate messaging could be conveyed. For example, it is not uncommon for students to arrive at the end of their medical school education and not know the differences between dependence and addiction, between misuse and abuse, and between tolerance and drug-seeking. It is also not uncommon for these same students to be unaware of many of these terms now being deemed stigmatizing and replaced with less judgmental terms— that words matter. These and other critically important related issues could be so much more effective if education became consistent, routinized, and promulgated. Educators are particularly important stakeholders indeed.

References

1. Dowell D, Haegerich TM, Chou R. CDC guideline for prescribing opioids for chronic pain — United States, 2016. MMWR Recomm Rep. 2016;65(RR-1):1–49.
2. U.S. Department of Health and Human Services. Pain management best practices inter-agency task force report: updates, gaps, inconsistencies, and recommendations. 2019, May. Retrieved from U. S. Department of Health and Human Services website: https://www.hhs.gov/ash/advisory-committees/pain/reports/index.html
3. Comerci G Jr, Katzman J, Duhigg D. Controlling the swing of the opioid pendulum. N Engl J Med. 2018;378(8):691–3.
4. Gourlay DL, Heit HA, Almahrezi A. Universal precautions in pain medicine: a rational approach to the treatment of chronic pain. Pain Med. 2005;6(2):107–12.
5. Dahl J, Joranson D. Relieving cancer pain/by June Dahl and David Joranson. World health. 1987, November 28–29. https://apps.who.int/iris/handle/10665/53413

6. Chou R, Fanciullo GJ, Fine PG, Adler JA, Ballantyne JC, Davies P, Donovan MI, Fishbain DA, Foley KM, Fudin J, Gilson AM, Kelter A, Mauskop A, O'Connor PG, Passik SD, Pasternak GW, Portenoy RK, Rich BA, Roberts RG, Todd KH, Miaskowski C. American Pain Society-American Academy of pain medicine opioids guidelines panel. Clinical guidelines for the use of chronic opioid therapy in chronic noncancer pain. J Pain. 2009;10(2):113–30.
7. Ault A. Opioid lawsuits push American Pain Society to Brink of Bankruptcy. Medscape News. 2019, May 29. https://www.medscape.com/viewarticle/913634. Accessed 20 June 2023.
8. McNamara D. American Pain Society officially shuttered. Medscape Medical News. 2019, July 02. https://www.medscape.com/viewarticle/915141#:~:text=It%27s%20official%20%E2%80%94%20the%20American%20Pain,diagnosis%20and%20management%20since%201978. Accessed 20 June 2023.
9. Gabay M. The federal controlled substances act: schedules and pharmacy registration. Hosp Pharm. 2013;48(6):473–4.
10. Katz NP, Adams EH, Benneyan JC, Birnbaum HG, Budman SH, Buzzeo RW, Carr DB, Cicero TJ, Gourlay D, Inciardi JA, Joranson DE, Kesslick J, Lande SD. Foundations of opioid risk management. Clin J Pain. 2007;23(2):103–18.
11. The Federation of State Medical Boards. Guidelines for the chronic use of opioid analgesics. 2017. https://www.fsmb.org/siteassets/advocacy/policies/opioid_guidelines_as_adopted_april-2017_final.pdf. https://www.fsmb.org/opioids/. Accessed 20 June 2023.
12. Mezei L, Murinson BB. Johns Hopkins pain curriculum development team. Pain education in North American medical schools. J Pain. 2011;12(12):1199–208.
13. Kress HG, Aldington D, Alon E, Coaccioli S, Collett B, Coluzzi F, Huygen F, Jaksch W, Kalso E, Kocot-Kępska M, Mangas AC, Ferri CM, Mavrocordatos P, Morlion B, Müller-Schwefe G, Nicolaou A, Hernández CP, Sichère P. A holistic approach to chronic pain management that involves all stakeholders: change is needed. Curr Med Res Opin. 2015;31(9):1743–54.
14. Office of National Drug Control Policy, President Barack Obama, The White House. National drug control strategy. 2011. https://obamawhitehouse.archives.gov/ondcp/2011-national-drug-control-strategy. Accessed 20 June 2023.
15. HHS recommends prescribing or co-prescribing naloxone to patients at high risk for an opioid overdose. U.S. Department of Health and Human Services. 2018, December 19. https://www.hhs.gov/opioids/treatment/overdose-response/index.html. Accessed 20 June 2023.

Challenges Facing Clinicians Treating Patients with Pain

6

The Challenge of How Pain Is Defined

Probably one of the greatest challenges facing clinicians who treat patients with pain today is the fact there is often a lack of consistency with respect to **how pain is defined**. When pain was designated the "5th vital sign" in 2000, in many people's minds pain became a number on a scale of 0–10, with 0 being no pain, and 10 being pain as bad as it could be. If it was documented in the medical record that a pain rating assessment was performed, it would be adequate to satisfy the "vital sign status." The result was that in many situations pain became a purely subjective symptom which could be easily documented and to some extent either discounted or something which could be improved based on a percentage basis of that number. For example, some postulated that they considered successful pain treatment to be a 33% reduction of pain rating, while others considered success to be a 2-point reduction in pain rating, and still others considering that successful pain treatment was "moving" the rating below a 5, regardless of the original number. Clearly, there was a need to standardize how pain was defined, which could then potentially improve satisfaction and pain treatment outcomes. As mentioned in Chap. 2, the International Association for the Study of Pain (IASP) redefined pain [1] in 2020 for the first time since 1979 with the intention of helping to create that higher level of conformity in defining pain among the medical community. Unfortunately, dissemination of this new definition was and continues to be relatively poor or completely absent. If you are unaware of this revised definition, it is a case in point.

The 2020 IASP definition defined pain as:

- An unpleasant **sensory and emotional experience** associated with, or resembling that associated with, actual or potential tissue damage—meaning that pain is an experience that involves not only what someone "feels" at a neurological level, but also what someone "feels" from an emotional perspective, and these feelings are not always equal in magnitude with respect to each other
- Something that is **always a personal experience** that is influenced to varying degrees by biological, psychological, and social factors—meaning that when

© The Author(s), under exclusive license to Springer Nature Switzerland AG 2024
K. L. Zacharoff, P. Migdal, *Pain, Drugs, and Ethics*,
https://doi.org/10.1007/978-3-031-63018-7_6

thinking about treatment planning, biological, psychological, and social factors need to be considered in terms of goals and expectations of that treatment plan

- Something that is *not* **synonymous with nociception**, with **pain and nociception being distinctly different phenomena**—meaning that pain cannot be inferred solely from activity in sensory neurons
- Something that is **a concept which individuals learn through their life experiences**—meaning that no two people may think of pain the same way
- An experience that **when it is reported by a patient should always be respected**—meaning that it should not be discounted, judged, or deemed unimportant
- Something that **typically serves an adaptive role**, but that **may have adverse effects on physical function and social and psychological well-being**
- Something that **can be expressed in many ways besides verbally**—meaning that someone who is unable to verbally communicate pain should not be deemed unable to experience pain

In the context of this revised definition, it is evident that pain is actually much more than purely a numerical rating on a scale of 0–10, and that a comprehensive pain assessment also requires functional, social, and psychological assessment as well—in a standardized and consistent way. This means that if a patient in Denver, Colorado, is assessed for pain, that assessment is no different than one that is performed in Bangor, Maine. This remains a significant challenge today as it is not uncommon for clinicians to assess pain and success of pain treatment differently even *within* a medical practice or healthcare system, let alone a community or region. The result is that often pain assessments, which are foundational elements of treatment planning, may be unstandardized, and that patient care may then be more likely to be variable, fragmented, and inconsistent in approach and outcomes. Ethically, what needs to happen is that promulgation of this information needs to take place, along with education about how to incorporate it into clinical practice, making it the standard of care.

The Challenge Presented by the Prevalence of Pain

Another challenge facing clinicians treating patients with pain today is the sheer number of people who suffer from it. As mentioned in Chapters 1 and 2, in 2011 the Institutes of Medicine (IOM) released a report titled ***Relieving Pain in America: A Blueprint for Transforming Prevention, Care, Education, and Research*** [2], which detailed the impact of pain on society from a quality-of-life and economic burden perspective in the United States estimating at the time that approximately 100 million people perspective in the United States. suffered from pain at any given time. This report was one of the first of its kind identifying that most of the pain care in the United States was provided by frontline practitioners in Primary Care settings, and *not* specialized pain treatment settings, such as pain clinics staffed by highly trained pain specialists who had much more education on the subject. More recently, in 2022 Yong et al. published an article [3] which updated the prevalence of chronic pain in adults in the United States. Their estimate was that more than 1 in 5 adults in the United States suffers from chronic pain (approximately 50.2 million), with approximately 10% of adults in the United States suffering "high-impact" chronic pain with disabling consequences. Additionally, they found that patients with chronic pain suffer significantly with respect to performance of activities of daily living, social engagement, and work-related limitations. They concluded that as mentioned above, comprehensive evaluations of pain should rely on individual impact, instead of simplistic pain ratings. Their estimation of annual economic impact due to lost productivity alone was between $299 and $335 billion.

Clinician-Level Challenges

From a clinical perspective, the high prevalence of pain translates to clinicians who may have had **little or no education about pain** treatment often shouldering the challenge of providing care to most patients with acute, subacute, and chronic pain which may frequently outnumber those patients they care for with diabetes, hypertension, and cancer combined. An analysis of opioid prescribing characteristics by Nora Volkow, the Director of the National Institute on Drug Abuse in 2011 [4] (which is likely to be similar to prescribing patterns today) reported that the majority of prescribers of opioid analgesics were general practitioners, such as family medicine physicians, and internists (in 2011, approximately 43% of all opioid prescriptions written). Most of these nonexpert clinicians often lacking more comprehensive education about opioid end up prescribing beyond awareness of implemented guidelines, system mandates, and dose restrictions, often leading to **variations in pain care**.

Additional clinical challenges clinicians often voice include that there is often **little time and resources** to devote an adequate amount of time to comprehensively assess patients with pain, with the other competing tasks they need to complete in the relatively short time that they have to spend with a patient, meaning that a detailed pain-related interview and deeper investigation into pain impact may not often be possible. This may result in treatment planning directed toward pain as a symptom, and not addressing pain from a pathophysiological perspectie which also considers the dynamic that exists between pain, mental health, and other stressors, such as social and economic factors.

Although not frequently considered, communication among healthcare professionals themselves is also often cited as a frequent challenge facing clinicians who treat patients with pain. This includes both inpatient, outpatient settings, and blended inpatient/outpatient settings when both exist for a given pain patient. Very often the electronic medical record may serve as the only vehicle of communication between healthcare professionals; one that is most often templated, not individualized, and in many ways not comparable or equally effective as verbal communication. Once again, time and resources are frequently reported to be significant barriers to interprofessional communication.

System-Level Challenges

Very often healthcare system-related issues can contribute to the challenges facing clinicians who manage patients with pain [5]. Most notable are **resource-limited or inconsistent processes** for managing patients with chronic pain. These challenges include not only inconsistent practices for assessing patients, but also for implementing treatment plans which provide care for patients consistently along the continuum of care, and the ability to effectively track pain treatment trajectories and outcomes. The current healthcare system climate is more often than not driven by and focused on opioid reduction strategies which may often overshadow goals for successful treatment. Additionally, when patients are deemed to require an assessment by a clinician with a higher level of expertise (such as a pain clinic), or to be transitioned from an acute care setting (such as the emergency department), to a chronic care setting, effective and consistent **policies and procedures for transitioning care** may be uncoordinated, fragmented, and even in some cases, unavailable or accessible (e.g., obtaining timely appointment at the pain clinic).

Patient-Level Challenges

The **complicated and individualized pain "experience"** may often present a challenge for clinicians. The fact that each patient's pain context is both subjective and unique has the potential to significantly influence both the assessment and treatment planning processes. **Patient goals and expectations of pain treatment** can vary as well, and although possibly challenging from a clinical perspective, they require calibration of them between clinician and patient to patient satisfaction. Additionally, another challenge to be considered is that **patients often present for pain treatment at different points during their clinical course**, which may include some period of self-treatment, treatment by other clinicians, or both.

Economic factors also can challenge the clinician to not only consider efficaciousness, but also to consider the patient's ability to shoulder the burden of cost including co-pays, deductibles, and other out-of-pocket expenses. For example, it is important to consider cost when working with the patient to formulate a pain treatment plan which incorporates over-the-counter medications, complementary and alternative therapies, or nonformulary pharmacologic agents. Treatments that are not likely to be initiated or continued because of the patient's inability to pay associated costs may challenge the clinician to look at other more realistic options or take the time and resources to obtain approval from the third-party payor (if there is one), which may further tax available clinic resources.

Regulatory Challenges

Fear of regulatory scrutiny is probably one of the biggest challenges a clinician faces today when making the determination that a patient is a candidate for an opioid analgesic trial, an adjustment (increase) in opioid dosing is required, or long-term opioid therapy is considered to be an appropriate possible course of action. It is important to note that there are many different guidelines for treating different painful conditions, and there is even variability in guideline-based recommendations for opioid prescribing. Nonexpert-level clinicians are frequently challenged with abiding by state medical board recommendations, as well as federal recommendations and requirements by the DEA, by the CDC, and the FDA to name a few. None have had a more chilling effect than the CDC Guideline for Prescribing Opioids for Chronic Pain published in 2016 [6]. In many cases, state medical boards adopted the CDC guidelines for nonexpert prescribing of opioids in their state for the sake of not "reinventing the wheel." After 2016, some clinicians increasingly reported that regulatory agency monitoring of opioid prescribing patterns obtained from the state PDMPs led to "threatening" communications from their state medical board, the DEA, or both which stated that the clinician's opioid prescribing patterns were determined to be outside the "normal levels" with respect to both numbers of opioid prescriptions written and dosages employed. This led many primary care clinicians to make the decision to not prescribe opioids to treat pain in their practice, or to severely restrict how opioids would be prescribed if they were continued, which many consider to be regulatory intention—to decrease the number of opioid prescriptions and amounts prescribed. In some cases, surgeons now only prescribe what is considered to be "enough" to manage pain in the immediate postsurgical period, recommending that the patient contact their primary care clinician for persistent pain in the absence of complications related to the surgery. This has further challenged those primary care clinicians already fearing retribution from regulators and feeling ethically conflicted about leaving the patient under on untreated.

The Challenge of Adherence

There are many different reasons why adherence to a pain treatment plan often presents itself as a significant challenge to clinicians treating patients with pain. **Nonbehavioral patient factors** include **individual patient demographics**, such as culture, upbringing, socioeconomic status, educational level, and household stability. **Behavioral patient factors** that may influence adherence include baseline level of physical activity, individual health interests, motivational levels, and willingness to actively participate in a pain treatment plan. **Clinician or health system-related factors** may influence patient adherence and include level of expertise (training), availability of resources, level of accessibility (e.g., ease of making an appointment), or recent receipt of a "warning notification" about opioid prescribing from a state or local regulatory agency, and stigmatizing policies and procedures. **Drug-related factors** which may influence level of patient adherence include how well the clinician is familiar with the patient and their individual life circumstances, which may potentially impact willingness to prescribe a controlled substance like an opioid analgesic, the clinician's prior experience with certain medications (such as opioids), the patient's past experiences with a medication, or past adherence history, and number of other medications being taken by the patient concurrently. **Pain-related factors** related to the clinician's experiences and the particular patient may influence patient adherence as well. These includes the presence or absence of and quality of trust and communication in the clinician-patient relationship, the past history of adherence to other pain treatment recommendations, the clinician's experience with patients with certain pain types (e.g., back pain, fibromyalgia, chronic headaches, etc.), the presence and number of medical and psychological comorbidities (e.g., anxiety, depression, obstructive sleep apnea, etc.), or how many other clinicians have been involved in attempts to provide treatment in the past, and the reasons responsible for those changes in care providers.

The Challenge of Scientific Evidence Basis

Clinicians treating patients with pain also often may find the controversy surrounding evidence basis of pain management (or lack of it) as a significant clinical challenge. This is particularly evident with respect to the **long-term use of opioid analgesics to treat chronic pain** along with the association between opioid prescribing and opioid-related overdose fatalities.

Even though as previously mentioned in earlier chapters that 2000–2010 was designated as the "Decade of Pain Control and Research" [7], answers to important questions about the use of opioid analgesics to treat chronic pain remain unanswered today. Anecdotally, there are many chronic pain sufferers who report that without opioids, their functional capacity would be significantly hampered. Alternatively, many experts opposing the use (or overuse) of opioids to treat chronic pain point to insufficient scientific evidence supporting the long-term use of opioids in this context is lacking to nonexistent [8]. This ongoing and often heated debate leaves clinicians feeling challenged about the best course of action to take for treating patients with chronic pain, especially along with the other challenges mentioned above. Additionally, many of the recommendations arguing against the use of opioids to treat chronic pain often do not offer substantial recommendations about alternative treatments that carry less risk than opioids to patients. In many cases, nonopioid medications are often proposed as alternatives to opioids, such as nonsteroidal anti-inflammatory drugs or acetaminophen. However, these medications are often relatively or absolutely contraindicated for many chronic pain patients, such as people over age 65, or those with hepatic impairment.

As mentioned above, regulators have implemented strategies and recommendations which are focused on decreasing opioid prescribing to help battle the increasing number of opioid-related opioid fatalities. The hypothesis was simple: increasing numbers of opioid prescriptions correlated directly with increasing numbers of opioid-related overdoses from 2000 and 2016, and the number of opioid prescriptions needed to decrease in order to stem the tide of overdose deaths. The challenge for clinicians was once again, how to decrease opioid prescribing but still maintain the moral responsibility to treat pain safely, compassionately, and effectively. A report from the American Medical Association in 2023 titled ***Physicians' actions to*** *help end the nation's drug-related overdose and death epidemic—and what still needs to be done* [9] found that even though opioid prescriptions decreased for the tenth consecutive year (a 49.4% decrease since 2012), overdose deaths continued to increase over that same 10-year period.

Few would question the value proposition of evidence-based practices to maintaining the highest level of quality of medical care, but these are just two examples of many gaps that exist in the scientific evidence base for treating pain which then leads to challenges for clinicians treating those patients.

The Challenges of Uncalibrated Goals and Expectations of Pain Treatment

When someone suffers an injury or event which results in acute pain, a well-defined and reproducible set of thoughts about goals, expectations, and concerns typically take place. This includes thinking about what needs to take place in order "to get better," or basically be "cured." Sometimes the approach may lend itself to a *RICE* approach, *R*est, *I*ce, *C*ompression, and *E*levation, other times, rest, rehabilitation, or even surgical intervention might be required. The point is that rarely does someone not extrapolate their clinical trajectory in terms of their goals and expectations of how their pain experience will be. Concerns may also likely exist regarding physical activity levels during this period, and when resumption of baseline levels of activity will likely occur. In these situations, challenges clinicians face usually involve answering questions, and "calibrating" goals and expectations based on past clinical experiences, individual patient characteristics, and patient needs. In a way, this is setting the stage for impressions about a shared vision for a successful treatment outcome, and not overly challenging.

When a patient's pain transitions from an acute pain experience to one of subacute or chronic pain, everything has the potential to change including the associated challenges both clinicians and patients face. In many cases, patients may use their own well-defined heuristics which apply to acute pain to formulate their goals and expectations about their subacute or chronic pain trajectory. In many circumstances, these might be inaccurate, but patients won't know that unless their healthcare professionals have specific discussions about them, helping them to understand and appropriately "recalibrate" their goals and expectations to be more realistic. Alternatively, it is also possible that the clinician's goals and expectations of the chronic pain trajectory may also be unrealistic or misrepresented. The intent might be to portray pain treatment and goals and expectations in a more positive light and to not be discouraging, instilling hope instead of painting an overly negative course and outcome. In some situations, clinicians may perceive the task of achieving calibrated realistic goals and expectations as a challenging and "difficult" discussion, and are sometimes inclined to avoid it altogether.

When there is incongruency between the patient's and clinician's goals and expectations of pain treatment, the potential for increased likelihood of patient dissatisfaction, adherence to the treatment plan, and unsuccessful treatment outcomes may exist. In many cases, particularly when treating chronic pain, the word "cure" should be avoided as it may increase the likelihood of unrealistically reachable goals. Amelioration or negotiation can often be much better terms to use, but it is important to remember that patients default to "cure." It can often be challenging for a clinician to navigate finding the appropriate calibrated balance between realistic goals and expectations and patient participation, motivation, and ultimately satisfaction, but it is critically important to achieve. Like most other clinician-patient encounters, communication and understanding are some of the most important pieces of the puzzle. Regardless of the pathology or diagnosis, the fact that the context of different patients is rarely ever the same, dictates that the goals and expectations of pain to treatment are not likely to be the same as well. As challenging as it might be, it is incumbent on the clinician to foster a mutual understanding of goals, expectations, and outcomes.

The Challenge of Mixed Messages

Since 2000, many other "pendulums" in addition to the "opioid pendulum" have been "swinging" and influencing pain care. Many "mixed messages" have been sent to clinicians about a variety of issues including but not limited to the "appropriate" prescribing of opioid analgesics, the moral imperative to treat people with pain, prescribed opioids' role in the overdose epidemic, and their relationship to substance use disorders, opioid use disorders, and addiction. Clinicians treating patients with pain have in many ways been caught in the crossfire of the tumultuous environment that persists today. Combined with sometimes competing, conflicting, and often shifting mixed-messaging, the impact on patient care has been a chilling roller coaster ride. In some cases, clinicians have attempted to adapt to these shifts as much as possible, and in other cases, as mentioned earlier in this chapter, the impact on patients has been chilling [10]. For some clinicians, the burden of balancing caring for patients with pain managed with long-term opioid analgesics with regulatory scrutiny became too great, and the decision was made to no longer provide prescriptions for them to those patients moving forward—effectively cutting patients off abruptly, even though they may have been managed with a stable regimen for a long time. For others, the decision has been made to just not prescribe opioids at all, regardless of the need or individual circumstances—leaving patients with no place to find someone to prescribe opioids to them, even if they were candidates for that treatment. And in other situations, patients have been informed that prescriptions for prescribed opioids would either no longer be available, forcibly tapered, or decreased significantly, each of these with consequences that further complicate how pain is managed, how patients with pain are perceived, and how patients in some cases feel stigmatized [11–13].

Clinicians have had the challenging task of figuring out how to comply with many "silver bullets" specifically targeted toward the "opioid crisis" which have significantly impacted the delivery of patient care. These include accessing state-managed Prescription Drug Monitoring Program databases (in some states mandated for each prescription of a controlled substance) to curb "drug-seeking," state mandates requiring a minimum amount of pain and substance use education for license registration renewal, the use of patient-provider agreements, and considering the co-prescription of naloxone whenever an opioid is prescribed to name a few. The associated challenges most often include some combination of balancing time, resources, regulations, guidelines, and, in many cases, frustration with accommodating what seems to be a continuing state of change and a sea of mixed messages.

These are just some of the examples of challenges that a clinician faces and must take into consideration when embarking on the complex task of treating patients with pain. They highlight the importance of education, standardized approaches, and patient-centered treatment planning that is directed toward both the biological and the biopsychosocial particularities of the patient with pain.

References

1. Raja SN, Carr DB, Cohen M, Finnerup NB, Flor H, Gibson S, Keefe FJ, Mogil JS, Ringkamp M, Sluka KA, Song XJ, Stevens B, Sullivan MD, Tutelman PR, Ushida T, Vader K. The revised International Association for the Study of Pain definition of pain: concepts, challenges, and compromises. Pain. 2020;161(9):1976–82.
2. Institute of Medicine (US). Committee on advancing pain research, care, and education. Relieving pain in America: a blueprint for transforming prevention, care, education, and research. Washington, DC: National Academies Press; 2011.
3. Yong RJ, Mullins PM, Bhattacharyya N. Prevalence of chronic pain among adults in the United States. Pain. 2022;163(2):e328–32.
4. Volkow ND, McLellan TA, Cotto JH, Karithanom M, Weiss SR. Characteristics of opioid prescriptions in 2009. JAMA. 2011;305(13):1299–301.
5. Polacek C, Christopher R, Mann M, Udall M, Craig T, Deminski M, Sathe NA. Healthcare professionals' perceptions of challenges to chronic pain management. Am J Manag Care. 2020;26(4):e135–9.
6. Dowell D, Haegerich TM, Chou R. CDC guideline for prescribing opioids for chronic pain – United States, 2016. MMWR Recomm Rep. 2016;65(1):1–49.
7. Brennan F. The US congressional "decade on pain control and research" 2001–2011: a review. J Pain Palliat Care Pharmacother. 2015;29(3):212–27.
8. Chou R, Turner JA, Devine EB, Hansen RN, Sullivan SD, Blazina I, Dana T, Bougatsos C, Deyo RA. The effectiveness and risks of long-term opioid therapy for chronic pain: a systematic review for a National Institutes of Health pathways to prevention workshop. Ann Intern Med. 2015;162(4):276–86.
9. The American Medical Association. Physicians' actions to help end the nation's drug-related overdose and death epidemic—and what still needs to be done. 2021, 2022, 2023. https://end-overdose-epidemic.org/. Accessed 22 June 2024.
10. Schmidt C. Experts worry about chilling effect of federal regulations on treating pain. J Natl Cancer Inst. 2005;97(8):554–5.
11. Benintendi A, Kosakowski S, Lagisetty P, Larochelle M, Bohnert ASB, Bazzi AR. "I felt like I had a scarlet letter": recurring experiences of structural stigma surrounding opioid tapers among patients with chronic, non-cancer pain. Drug Alcohol Depend. 2021;222:108664.
12. Slade SC, Molloy E, Keating JL. Stigma experienced by people with nonspecific chronic low back pain: a qualitative study. Pain Med. 2009;10(1):143–54.
13. Waugh OC, Byrne DG, Nicholas MK. Internalized stigma in people living with chronic pain. J Pain. 2014;15(5):550.e1–10.

Dilemmas Surrounding Opioid Analgesics and the Treatment of Pain

7

When we examine the relationship between opioid analgesics and their utility in the treatment of pain, it should not be surprising that many clinical dilemmas exist. In fact, it is possible that there may be no greater controversy associated with the treatment of pain than the use of these drugs as part of a treatment plan and ethical issues related to their use. In fact, in many cases it can often be virtually impossible to discuss pain and its management without some inclusion of, or reference to, opioids including whether they should *ever* be used to treat pain, and the relationship of prescribed opioid analgesics to the overdose crisis that exists in the United States today. This often results in the development of several dilemmas for clinicians *and* patients because pain treatment has so often been associated with opioid prescribing in the past and present, and, in some ways, their relationship is inseparable both cognitively and pre-cognitively. Additionally, virtually every other stakeholder in the world of pain management, from policymakers to pharmaceutical companies face dilemmas related to this topic as well. Even though it may seem as if the challenges we face today regarding the overdose epidemic and opioids are considered to be (fairly) recent occurrences, in fact, little if anything about this relationship is "new." Opioid analgesics and issues surrounding "unhealthy" use of them (e.g., use for nonmedical purposes) are thousands of years old, and controversies about their relationship are equally as old. More about this will be discussed in a later chapter about the "opioid" epidemic.

The Decision to Use of Opioid Analgesics to Treat Pain

It is important to remember that opioid analgesics *do not* directly have a therapeutic effect on the pathophysiologic cause(s) of pain. A good analogy might be to think of them as earplugs which are employed to mute the "noise" of pain—but is important to remember that these "earplugs" are not doing anything to stop the source of the "noise"; these earplugs typically work to dampen the perception of pain, modifying pain severity or even in some cases by completely "blocking it out." Opioids

© The Author(s), under exclusive license to Springer Nature Switzerland AG 2024
K. L. Zacharoff, P. Migdal, *Pain, Drugs, and Ethics*,
https://doi.org/10.1007/978-3-031-63018-7_7

work to help "mute" pain in most cases, without impacting the cause of pain. Certainly, it could be argued that secondarily opioids could actually be considered to be therapeutic in a variety of ways, including assisting in the ability to rest and recover, helping to allow for increased function in the face of pain which would normally prohibit it, or by facilitating participation in rehabilitative activities such as physical therapy to name a few. In this regard, they indeed *do* have some therapeutic role, but for the purposes of this discussion think of them as being different in their therapeutic value compared to other commonly employed medications which have distinct therapeutic effects such as antibiotics, beta blockers, diuretics, blood thinners, etc.

This lack of clarity about the therapeutic profile of opioid analgesics sets the stage for one dilemma surrounding their use to treat pain—**whether or not there is truly a benefit for their use for this purpose.** Few would argue that in the most acute and *objectively* painful situations (i.e., those which have an identifiable cause or etiology) such as postsurgical pain or pain associated with an acute injury, opioid analgesics are likely to play a significantly important role in helping to compassionately alleviate pain and associated suffering. Many would also advocate for their use in other acute situations that are typically known to be severely painful (such as renal colic) as well. But one thing related to this construct which has changed over the past 20+ years is that today there is a very vocal and passionate debate about the rationale for what period of time they should be used to treat acute pain, and whether or not they should be used in most cases at all. One recurring underlying theme in this particular debate involves whether opioids have been overutilized in the past as first-line pain relievers for acute pain, resulting from their being overprescribed, in larger quantities than likely needed in the majority of situations. Most would agree that looking back at the period of "liberal" opioid prescribing (the late 1990s and early 2000s), the answer to the question of overutilization is unquestionably *affirmative*. At the time, it was quite common for opioids to be prescribed for a prolonged (or even undefined) periods of time, with dosages that were in many cases arbitrary, and a recommended frequency of dosing that ranged from around-the-clock to as-needed with little other clinical guidance. But it is also important to remember that during this same period, clinicians (most often doctors) were in many cases criticized and even in some cases successfully litigated for undertreating someone's pain, alleviating their suffering, or neglecting to treat pain entirely. These lawsuits and criticisms were sometimes initiated by patients themselves, and in other cases by family members who did not want to see their loved ones left inadequately or untreated for pain and suffering. Reactively, doctors responded with their "prescription pads" prescribing pain relievers liberally in an attempt to respond to these claims both morally and ethically. Additionally, during this period of liberal prescribing, in many cases opioids were prescribed in quantities and frequency with the intention of achieving a variety of different goals. This included making sure that the patient had "enough" medication prescribed to them to ensure that they would not deplete their supply during times of "off hours" when the prescribing clinician was unavailable and the analgesic need persisted, such as evenings, weekends, etc. Further, there was often lack of clarity about how long the opioid should be taken once it was started, often with little or no instruction about "they should only be taken until they were no longer needed." One might expect that there were many situations where there was a high level of variability in that regard, with some patients who would stop the opioids when their pain was tolerable or alleviated, and other situations where patients who for a variety of reasons continued to take the opioids for a longer period of time than expected, and needed continuing refills, which in many cases were given to them by default or without any pain assessment beyond a subjective, self-reported numerical pain rating. What may have been critically missing from the clinical equation at the time was the ability to mutually identify *with the patient,* a definitive value proposition that considered the risk of continued opioid use versus the benefit of their use in the face of persistent pain or continued prescribing. Again, it is important to keep in mind the fact that in many of these situations, the prescribers were largely clinicians who may have received little or virtually no education about pain, its treatment, and associated substance use or aberrant drug-related behaviors related to opioids or other controlled substances.

It is important to remember that much of the battle for people with pain to be adequately treated during this period was led by the American Cancer Society, whose mission was to ensure that patients with cancer and cancer-related pain were afforded the moral and ethical pain treatment they deserved. Coinciding with the designation of pain as the 5th Vital Sign, this provided fertile ground to spill over to include anyone with a non cancer pain-related complaint considered to be valid. Again it is important to reiterate that this took place with little or no education being provided to clinicians about how to assess and treat pain appropriately, safely, and effectively, and virtually no education about aberrant drug-related behaviors and addiction. Additionally, little to no education was provided to patients and caregivers about the potential risks of opioids (beyond opioid-related side effects such as constipation) compared to their potential benefits. To further complicate matters, aggressive marketing campaigns by opioid manufacturers became commonplace to "help" better manage patients with pain. It seemed as if everything at the time was directed toward increased prescribing of opioids to be the answer to pain and related suffering.

On the heels of this period of liberal prescribing, several regulatory efforts, including the implementation of state-managed controlled prescription database programs (prescription drug monitoring programs or PDMPs), increased availability of naloxone to people at increased risk of overdose, the focus being on decreasing the number of opioid prescriptions. The most notable effort for this change was likely the 2016 CDC Guidelines for Prescribing Opioids for the Management of Chronic Pain [1]. In a way, this helped to fuel the dilemma associated with opioid prescribing because from a regulatory perspective, it seemed as if the only answer to the ever-increasing number of drug-related overdose deaths was to decrease the number of opioid prescriptions written, the duration for which they were prescribed, and the dosages provided in all but the most expert levels of clinical pain practice.

Inconsistent Terminology

Words make a difference, and being labeled has consequences. It is unethical to label someone or something in a demeaning way, but it is also realistic to acknowledge that whether cognitively or pre-cognitively, being labeled happens to people with pain frequently. Patients with chronic pain and those with chronic pain treated with long-term opioid therapy often report that one or both of these factors has led to them being labeled, judged, and stigmatized [2]. Notably, in these instances patients have experienced these behaviors from many sources including friends, family members, co-workers, and healthcare professionals. Inconsistent terminology has the potential to further contribute to this stigmatization, ultimately presenting more challenges for patients with pain *and* clinicians treating them with opioid analgesics, even when they may be appropriate components of a pain treatment plan.

For example, terms like misuse and abuse of medications have frequently been used interchangeably to describe the same situation as if they meant the same thing. Additionally, there has been frequent and often inaccurate substitution of the term dependence for addiction [3]. In the past, **misuse** referred to the use of a medication for *medical* purposes in a way other than as prescribed. For example, if someone was prescribed an opioid medication for pain treatment, and they either took greater amounts than prescribed, or took it more frequently than prescribed, it was referred to as *misuse*—using the medication for the intended reason, just not in the way directed. This is quite different than **abuse**, which referred to either *any* illicit use of a drug or substance, and/or the intentional self-administration of a medication or substance (including alcohol) for a *nonmedical* purposes (such as to get "high"). Both terms are being used less frequently today, as they are considered by many to be stigmatizing and are slowly being replaced with nonstigmatizing language such as "unhealthy use," but that change has been slow, and, in the absence of education, may potentially cause even more confusion for everyone involved. The point is that if someone were considered to be *misusing* their opioid medication, it is quite a different situation than if they were *abusing* it. Unfortunately, in many cases, including pieces in the mainstream media, articles in the medical literature, curricula in educational programs, and even regulatory agency policy statements, recommendations, and guidelines, these terms have been used as if they are synonymous with each other, which they are not. This has been, and continues to be, a dilemma particularly with respect to opioid analgesics, because of the significant difference in definitions of the two terms, and the potential implications of their use inappropriately. For example, someone who may be increasing their intake of opioids to better attempt to control their pain (misusing their opioid medication) is very different from someone who is using them to get "high" (abusing their opioid medication). It is not difficult to imagine how someone being mislabeled as an abuser could create several unintended consequences and how misinterpreting the differences between misuse and abuse creates many dilemmas for virtually all stakeholders involved.

Another dilemma with respect to inconsistent terminology involving opioid analgesic therapy is the frequent synonymous use of **dependence** and **addiction**. In some cases, the differences or similarities between dependence and addiction may be misunderstood by patients, clinicians, and other stakeholders, with the resulting potential clinical implications being significant. For example, it is not uncommon for a patient recommended an opioid analgesic to inquire about concern related to the likelihood of them becoming "addicted" to it. Depending on how someone defines addiction will likely impact the answer to what can often be a relatively simple answer to that question—whether or not the person answering that question considers dependence and addiction to be the same. If the question is truly about dependence, then the answer may likely be that after some period of time dependence is likely. If addiction is considered to be distinctly different from dependence, the answer may likely be that addiction is possible, but statistically unlikely in the absence of other risk factors for its development. This could be instead used as a teaching moment to help educate the patient about the differences between dependence and addiction: that **physical dependence** is a natural state of adaptation when opioids are prescribed for any time longer than a very brief period, and that it is not uncommon or abnormal for their bodies to become "used to" or "dependent" on them. This dependence may in many cases manifest itself with the development of withdrawal or withdrawal-like symptoms if they are abruptly discontinued. Unfortunately, to many patients and clinicians, dependence is often used interchangeably with addiction. If the question about concern of developing addiction is answered affirmatively because of a lack of clarity about the differences between addiction and dependence are defined, one consequence might be refusal of the use of opioids because of fear of becoming addicted to them, despite the fact that they might have potentially had a significantly positive role in the pain treatment plan and functional capacity. In fact, it is not uncommon for even postsurgical patients to refuse an opioid because of fears associated with developing addiction even after a short course of opioid exposure, even though their fears may be unfounded because of misunderstanding the difference between addiction and dependence. **Addiction** is a primary, chronic neurobiological disease with several factors involved in its development and manifestation, including genetic, psychological, and environmental ones. Comparatively, behavioral characteristics of addiction include impaired control over use, compulsive use, continued use despite harm, and craving for use. If someone with an addiction to an opioid abruptly discontinues them, they may likely develop withdrawal or withdrawal like symptoms, but that is where the similarities between physical dependence addiction end. Potentially further confusing this issue is that **psychological dependence**, which is generally meant to describe the emotional and mental processes that are associated with the development of, and/or recovery from, a substance use disorder or addiction, is frequently shortened by healthcare profession-als to "dependence," with the intention of referring to addiction or substance use dis-order. This can further contribute to the inconsistency in interpretation and understanding, which may present itself as a significant dilemma for patients and cli-nicians alike. What we say and what we mean when we say it matter, and it is very important for there to be consistency of terminology and clear understanding of the terms we use and the messages we are trying to convey. Often, like many other times mentioned in this text, education is a critical piece of the puzzle to mitigate the lack of consistency in terminology surrounding opioid analgesia, dependence, and addiction.

Mixed Messaging

As mentioned earlier in this chapter, what has become apparent in recent years is that there are more questions about the risks and benefits of opioid use beyond the shortest possible length of time, or, in some cases, their use to treat pain at all. This contradicts clinical paradigms where opioids have been frequently utilized to treat subacute or chronic painful conditions. Since the recognition of the relationship between opioid prescribing and the overdose crisis, there has been a concerted effort by regulatory and governmental agencies to decrease the frequency and number of opioid analgesics prescribed to patients as a major strategy to stem the tide of increasing overdose fatalities in the United States. As mentioned in Chap. 6, a recent report by the American Medical Association in a 2023 titled *Physicians' Actions to Help End the Nation's Drug-Related Overdose and Death Epidemic —and What Still Needs to be Done* [4] detailed the "success of these efforts, with opioid prescriptions decreasing 49.4% from 257.9 million to 131.9 million between 2012 and 2022. In fact, this was the lowest number of prescriptions for opioids in the United States since 1993, long before the overdose epidemic. What must be considered is the clinical impact that this opioid-diminishing strategy has had on prescribers, patients, caregivers, and society overall. In many cases, consequences of these initiatives have included decreased levels of clinician willingness to prescribe opioid analgesics to any patients (even if opioids might have been previously considered to be an appropriate component of a pain treatment plan), scrutiny of those clinicians who prescribe them with higher frequency, duration, or quantities, than their peers, and ultimately decreased access for patients who were on opioid analgesic therapy on a long-term basis or who needed them in order to maintain functionality, quality of life, or both. In some cases, there has been significant concern that patients who encounter diminished access to opioid prescriptions might seek to secure them from illicit channel of distribution in order to maintain their baseline quality of life, potentially exposing them to increased risk instead. Research and commentaries are beginning to appear in the scientific literature and even in the mainstream media about the untended harms of either forcibly tapering or abruptly discontinuing opioids for someone on stable long-term opioid therapy [5–7]. The release of the 2016 CDC guidelines for prescribing opioids for the treatment of chronic non cancer pain [1] is an illustrative example of how mixed messaging created dilemmas for patients and clinicians alike. Within 3 years of their release, an editorial was published in the *New England Journal of Medicine* titled *No Shortcuts to Safer Opioid Prescribing* [8] detailing how often-inconsistent practices and policies followed the CDC Guideline release, including what these authors referred to as "*inflexible application of recommended dosage and duration thresholds, policies which encouraged hard limits and abrupt opioid tapering, sudden discontinuation, or dismissal of patients from a physician's practice.*" Additionally, this commentary referred to "misapplication" of the CDC Guidelines to patient populations outside the intended scope. While the intention of this editorial was to clarify how the guidelines were intended to be used, in many cases it highlighted dilemmas which exist for patients and clinicians in today's medical environment as a result of them. For some, these guidelines only created further conflict for clinicians particularly about the "right" and "wrong" thing to do with respect to opioid prescribing. This translated to patients in many cases not knowing what to do when faced with a clinician no longer willing to continue to prescribe an opioid to them, regardless of whether they were being managed safely and successfully or not. In 2022, the CDC announced that it was undertaking a process for revising the 2016 Guidelines with the intention to make them clearer, more patient-centric, and less like a mandate. Many pain advocates pointed out that to some degree the "damage" had already been done, that it was "too little, too late," and that reversing the impact of the 2016 guidelines would be more challenging than anticipated. In their commentary related to the draft version of the revised 2022 CDC Guidelines, the American Medical Association commented that there would need to be a significant effort to "undo" the messaging in the original guidelines, and that it would not likely be easy, presenting another dilemma for patients and clinicians regarding the use of opioid analgesics to treat pain.

It is important to consider that virtually no pain treatment approach is without some degree of inherent risk. Non opioid pharmacologic approaches have been suggested to clinicians as alternatives to opioids for treating chronic pain, including the use of nonsteroidal anti-inflammatory drugs (NSAIDs), acetaminophen, and other nonopioid medications or interventional treatments. For example, NSAIDs and acetaminophen both can have significant risks associated with their use, especially on a chronic basis, and for many patients they may be relatively or absolutely contraindicated for the treatment of pain. One illustrative example is the consideration of using NSAIDs for patients 65 years of age or older, or patients who have a history of cardiovascular disease. Because of associated adverse effects and the risk/benefit profile of NSAIDs in this patient population, these medications may not necessarily be the safest pharmacologic choice for treating pain in these patients. In certain cases, they may be relatively *or* absolutely contraindicated for use. Similar risks exist for the prolonged use of acetaminophen products in patients with liver dysfunction. With respect to other adjunctive (or adjuvant) pharmacologic nonopioid medications, which are defined as drugs that do not contain acetaminophen and those not classified as nonsteroidal anti-inflammatory or opioid agents, such as anti depressants or anti convulsants, in some instances their adverse effect or drug-drug interaction profile may negatively affect the calculus of risk versus benefit. Additionally, in some cases, non medical use of these agents has the potential to impact risk as well. Interventional treatments, although often quite effective, have risk associated with them as well, including potential adverse effects related to steroidal medications which might often be employed, and limited long-term benefit to name a few.

Non pharmacologic approaches have been suggested as alternatives to opioid therapy as well, including physical therapy, acupuncture, and other complementary techniques such as cognitive behavioral therapy. Without question, these approaches play a significant role in a multimodal and multidisciplinary pain treatment plan. However, it is also important to consider that in some cases, these treatments may be limited by several factors including availability, access, insurance coverage (if *there is* insurance coverage), and the patient's ability to pay out-of-pocket if necessary.

It is important to remember that in most cases, the least costly (economic cost), and in many cases the most economically attractive component of a chronic pain treatment plan to payers may in fact be opioid analgesics. Payers are often most interested in what will ultimately be the least expensive course of action. Clinicians are often challenged with unreimbursed resource expenditures related to the determination of "what is covered and what is not," and this is a common dilemma they face. Patients are often most interested in treatment choices that are the least likely to "challenge" them from an economic perspective. Taken together, this translates to the fact that economic issues may exert significant force on the dilemma that both patients and clinicians face with respect to the utilization of opioids or other pain treatment approaches. In the late 1990s and early 2000s it was common practice to prescribe larger quantities of opioids than what would be anticipated to be needed to precisely avoid these kinds of situations.

Fear of Regulatory Scrutiny

Fear of regulatory scrutiny against clinicians who utilize opioid analgesics as a component of a pain treatment plan when appropriate is real, and often presents a major dilemma for clinicians and patients. Since the relationship of what many consider to be "liberal prescribing" of opioids was first identified to be associated with a direct increase of unintentional drug-related overdose fatalities, regulatory agencies have implemented many tactics and strategies to do a variety of things to intervene, such as increasing education of clinicians and patients, promulgation of tools to promote responsible prescribing, increased availability of naloxone, etc. It is important to consider all the stakeholders who play a role as regulators in this regard. These include state medical boards, federal agencies such as the FDA, the CDC, and the DEA, but it is also important to include other stakeholders who might not often be considered as regulators like insurers and pharmacy boards, who may also play a significant role in discouraging opioid prescribing. But most clinicians likely would likely say that they have faced a dilemma associated with one over-arching goal—**the intent by regulatory agencies to decrease the number of opioid prescriptions and the quantities of opioids prescribed**. Whether it was the result of publications in the scientific literature, pieces in the mainstream media, or language used in clinical practice guidelines such as those issued by the CDC in 2016, clinicians wanted to avoid being "flagged" by a regulatory agency or state medical board as someone who prescribed opioids "inappropriately." The word **risk** started to take on a new meaning, no longer just referring to risk of adverse effects or aberrant drug-related use. Clinicians became fearful of the **risk of regulatory scrutiny**, and patients became fearful about the **risk of losing access to their critically important pain medications**. It had become clear that regulatory agencies were "watching," and clinicians indeed knew that they were being watched.

Every state (along with the District of Columbia) in the country now has a state-managed database program designed to capture data regarding prescribing of controlled substances. These databases are referred to as **Prescription Drug**

Monitoring Programs (PDMPs). One of the key intended purposes of these data-capturing programs is **risk mitigation**, enabling clinicians to have the ability to access data to capture information about controlled substances prescribed to their patients to better inform clinical decision-making. For example, PDMPs could help to determine whether patients might be obtaining multiple prescriptions for controlled substances, such as opioid analgesics from other clinicians for many reasons, including aberrant use, addictive behaviors, or even diversion for profit. This has been referred to in the past in many ways, including "drug-seeking behavior(s)," "doctor shopping," medication-seeking, etc. The specific rules and regulations governing the PDMP use vary from state to state, with some states mandating that the database be checked prior to prescribing any controlled substance, and others urging their use on a voluntary basis. In addition to providing access to this information to clinicians, this data also allows for clinicians to be aware of other medications being prescribed to patients by other clinicians which could be potentially harmful with respect to drug-drug interactions, possible potentiation of adverse effects, or even metabolic competition (harmful polypharmacy).

But another important function of PDMPs as data warehouses is to provide information to local and federal regulatory agencies (such as the state medical board, the DEA, etc.) about clinician-level controlled substance (including opioid analgesics) prescribing practices and patterns which might be considered to be "high-risk." These patterns could include falling outside of the "normal" range of frequency of prescribing, and "excessively high" prescribed quantities and or dosages. This type of data analysis is often derived through comparison to prescribing patterns of other similar-specialty clinicians in a given geographic area or region.

The implementation of PDMPs has long been considered to be a key opioid risk minimization strategy by virtually all regulatory agencies to promote safe practices in an effort to combat the overdose crisis our country faces, yet controversy exists with respect to their utility in this regard [9]. Unfortunately, clinicians and patients may face several dilemmas resulting from the implementation of PDMPs and the controversies surrounding them. One dilemma is that with almost every state having its own database, sharing of information across state lines has been inconsistent, and in some cases even nonexistent. Progress has been made with respect to this issue, but even though cooperatives do exist between some neighboring states, many often question why the database is not national, with information sharing seamlessly across the entire country. Probably the single biggest dilemma facing clinicians with respect to PDMPs is concern about the likely result of radical changes in opioid prescribing practices due to fear of regulatory scrutiny from the agencies having access to this data. This could then have a ripple effect of contributing to a patient's dilemma of either having to look for another means of obtaining their prescription, or having their pain go under- or untreated, with resulting potential consequences ranging from anxiety to mental health related issues, and in some cases suicide [7]. Another associated dilemma is the impact that PDMPs have had on the practice of medicine, with clinicians often voicing concern about PDMP impact on their autonomy as healthcare professionals, in some cases a local deficit of clinicians with a higher level of expertise (i.e., pain specialists) for potential referral, the time and resources necessary to comply with checking the PDMPs, poor integration with electronic medical record systems, and access to timely (real-time) data provided by PDMPs to name a few. Few would question that programs such as PDMPs play a significant role in safe and appropriate opioid and other controlled substance prescribing practices. But research, care, effort, and coordination are likely steps which need to be taken so PDMPs aren't solely perceived as tools that promote further fears of regulatory scrutiny.

Risks Related to Opioids

Up until the time when the drug overdose epidemic in the United States became apparent, the clinical definition of the term "**opioid risk**" meant something different than it does today. Until that point, opioid risk most often referred to adverse effects related to opioid administration. The list of those adverse effects included constipation, nausea, vomiting, itching, drowsiness, and **respiratory depression**. Respiratory depression was considered to be the most serious of these adverse effects, and if left unidentified and/or untreated, it could lead to fatal consequences. People who were determined to be at increased risk of developing opioid-induced respiratory depression were either considered to be poor candidates for their use or were informed that they would need to be monitored closely for this potentially serious side effect. This often included a variety of patients at increased risk, including those who had a history of some type of respiratory illness, people with sleep apnea, or people who were morbidly obese. Additionally, virtually all people who were treated with opioids were considered to be at increased risk of developing **constipation**, particularly those who were postsurgical, had a diagnosis of cancer, or had a prior history of chronic constipation, and were in many cases treated with a prophylactic regimen including laxatives, stool softeners, etc. Regardless of the specific adverse effect, the risk/benefit analysis for opioid therapy was considered, presented to the patient, and/or caregiver as part of the informed consent process, and initiated if the analysis was favorable or if no other safe and effective options for pain treatment existed. The decision involved patient-level risk and was generally between patient and prescriber.

Today, the term "opioid risk" is frequently used to refer to describing someone's risk of either portraying an aberrant drug-related behavior (such as abuse, misuse, or diversion), becoming dependent (*psychologically* dependent), or addicted to them. The mainstream media has adopted this definition of opioid risk as well in the context of prescription opioids and their role in contributing to the overdose epidemic. This modern-day interpretation has been adopted by virtually all stakeholders, and most commonly refers to a determination based on the clinician's ability to assess "opioid risk" when an opioid is considered to be an appropriate component of a pain treatment plan. Regulatory agencies, such as the U.S. Food and Drug Administration (FDA) use this term in the context of their evaluation of opioid safety and efficacy, which then directly impacts pharmaceutical companies and marketing of their opioid products. In fact, when a pharmaceutical company applies to the FDA for approval of an opioid medication, often the application must include a *risk management plan* which specifically details steps that the company will take to mitigate this "opioid risk" to not only the patient, but also to members of the patient's household, the patient's community, and society at large. In some cases, this plan may need to be more detailed, if the FDA determines that the potential risk for aberrant use or addiction is significant enough to warrant it. These more detailed risk management plans are called **Risk Evaluation and Mitigation Strategies, or REMS** [10]. The FDA now requires a REMS for <u>all</u> formulations of opioid analgesics [11], stating that "under the conditions specified in this opioid REMS, with providers of opioid analgesics (e.g., pharmacists) and healthcare professionals who prescribe them and provide care to patients and their caregivers strongly encouraged to do all of the following:" (1) educate themselves about safe and appropriate opioid prescribing, (2) counsel patients and caregivers about safe opioid use, including storage and disposal, (3) stress the importance of reading and understanding the medication guide provided when opioids are dispensed, and (4) to consider using tools to improve patient, household, and community safety, such as a Patient-Provider Agreement (PPA), and validated opioid risk assessment instruments that may assist in predicting the likelihood of aberrant behaviors and/or addiction.

In some ways, the common opioid-related adverse effects which affect most patients to whom they are administered have been somewhat overshadowed by the overdose crisis and the regulatory concerns associated with it. It is important to understand that *both* definitions of "opioid risk" need to be considered when opioids are considered to treat pain.

The Opioid "Pendulum"

To most clinicians, the term "opioid pendulum" [12] refers to the dramatic transition with respect to prescribing patterns of opioid analgesics in the United States over the past 20+ years, often associated with the designation of pain as the 5th vital sign in 2000. As mentioned many times throughout the course of this book, given the fact that most frontline practitioners who typically shoulder the majority of patients with pain-related complaints may have had little to no education about pain management, substance use, or opioids beyond basic pharmacology, the stage seemed to have been set for liberal prescribing of opioids to best treat patients suffering from pain. Making pain something that needed to be assessed as a "vital sign" meant that something needed to be done to treat it once it was identified. Add to that the fact that in the late 1990s clinicians were successfully being litigated, reprimanded, or both for the undertreatment or complete inattention to pain as a condition warranting definitive treatment. Of course, all of this taking place in the presence of what is now considered by many to be "overly aggressive" and sometimes inaccurate marketing of opioid analgesics by pharmaceutical companies who manufactured them and minimized the risks associated with them—most notably addiction.

If we look back at the first decade after 2000, it is probably fair to say that the opioid pendulum moved in the direction of liberal opioid prescribing [13] for pain-related complaints across the entire country. Patients often treated themselves (and still continue to do so) with over-the-counter medications like acetaminophen and NSAIDs (e.g., ibuprofen) prior to seeking medical attention, and felt entitled to something "stronger" for their pain, and as mentioned previously prescribers responded with their prescription pads. In fact, around 2010, opioid analgesics became *the* most commonly prescribed class of medications in the United States. This was not surprising at the time, since pain was (and continues to be) the single most common reason that patients sought medical attention. By 2010, many referred to the concurrent trends of increasing prescribing of opioids and opioid-related overdoses and overdose fatalities as being intimately related, including the Office of National Drug Control Policy and the White House. In its 2011 report and action plan, the Office of the President of the United States titled *EPIDEMIC: Responding to America's Prescription Drug Abuse Crisis* [14] underscored the relationship between prescribed opioids and overdose deaths. This was the beginning of the "swing" in the direction away from liberal opioid prescribing. In fact, by the time that the *CDC Guidelines for Opioid Prescribing Opioids for Chronic Pain* were released in 2016, virtually every regulatory agency in the United States was aligned in their missions to stem the tide of overdose fatalities by decreasing the number of opioid prescriptions and amounts prescribed. The pendulum started to swing in the opposite direction: less prescribing of opioids and more scrutiny of clinicians who continued to prescribe them liberally, or as some agencies such as the Federation of State Medical Boards stated, "inappropriately."

In some cases, the effect of this pendulum-like phenomenon of opioid prescribing was chilling, with some clinicians, clinician practices, and even in some cases clinics and institutions adopting "no opioid prescribing" policies. In other cases, state medical boards adopted limits recommended in the 2016 CDC Guidelines for how much and for what duration opioids could be prescribed by "nonexpert" clinicians, such as frontline practitioners in primary care and internal medicine settings. Data obtained from the PDMPs would then be able to identify clinicians who deviated from the recommendations for these limits. Some states such as California, implemented very aggressive policies like the "Death Certificate Project" [15] which contributed to making clinicians fearful of scrutiny if opioids were prescribed to any patient. In some states, even the names of their PDMPs evoked fear of reprisal, with the California PDMP named the *California Controlled Substance Utilization Review and Evaluation System* (CURES). In New York, the PDMP database was named ISTOP, the Internet System for Tracking Over-Prescribing, implying that the purpose of the database was directed toward clinician prescribing practices.

The chilling effect ultimately had the most impact on people with pain being assessed and/or treated with opioid analgesics for their pain, who in many cases were unexpectedly faced with clinicians unwilling to prescribe pain medications or to continue dosages previously used for fear of regulatory repercussions. At this point, many clinicians deemed the "risk" of prescribing opioids from a regulatory scrutiny perspective to be too high. Challenges for these patients included being forced to somehow deal with this sudden transition with little or no guidance, associated withdrawal symptoms due to physiologic dependence, and finding someone who would be willing to continue prescribing the opioid medication in a timely manner. Alternatively, a potential societal dilemma was the fear of some of these patients would turn to illicit sources to supply their longstanding opioid therapy and have an increased risk of being potentially exposed to counterfeit preparations tainted with illicit fentanyl, which could be fatal.

Lack of Consensus and Scientific Evidence for Long-Term Opioid Therapy

The term "best practices" in medicine typically refers to practices that have an evidence-basis. With respect to most common medical conditions and their treatment, it is generally not difficult to develop consensus on the basis of available scientific evidence and derive value in terms of delivering care on the basis of these "best practices." There have been situations where the evidence basis changes due to new research, developments, etc., but it is fair to say that when there are available evidence-based treatment recommendations, they are most often considered to be the most desirable approach to care, and there is often little to no controversy in that regard.

However, when it comes to consensus and scientific evidence for the long-term use of opioids in the management of chronic pain, things do not tend to fit into that mold. It is not difficult to find large numbers of patients with pain who report that opioid analgesics prescribed to them for chronic pain conditions on a long-term basis has been critically important to their ability to maintain some degree of functional capacity with respect to daily activities, including work, social interaction, exercise, etc. It is also not difficult to find many who challenge the use of long-term opioid therapy argue that the scientific evidence basis for opioid therapy longer than 6 months is lacking, and that the risk of addiction, overdose, and substance use disorder may outweigh potential benefits. In fact, ever since the association between the opioid prescribing and the increase in drug-related overdoses and fatalities was identified, there has been a widespread call for scientific research to answer the question of long-term opioid efficacy and safety. Unfortunately, for clinicians, patients, and other stakeholders, available research is relatively sparse and often conflicting, either pointing to evidence supporting the benefits if a comprehensive and rational risk/benefit analysis is performed [16], or pointing to evidence showing little or no benefit, and in some cases referring to potential harm including increased risk of aberrant drug-related behaviors and addiction [17].

The end result of this lack of consensus and scientific evidence often presents a number of dilemmas for both clinicians and the patients with chronic pain that they are called upon to treat. The most notable challenge is a relative lack of consistency with respect to assessment, treatment plan formation, and decision-making surrounding the possible utility of long-term opioid therapy. As mentioned previously, this lack of consistency may exist within a given practice setting (with different clinicians expressing different opinions), clinic, institution, healthcare system, or even at the payer level, often resulting in confusion and inconsistent continuity of care. Given all of the other challenges regarding the use of opioid analgesics mentioned above, in many cases people just do not have a consistent way to know how to arrive at the most appropriate course of action. To further complicate matters, with all the controversy surrounding long-term opioid therapy, there is often very little discussion about alternative approaches. Generalized statements supporting the use of nonopioid approaches, non pharmacological approaches, and complementary and alternative treatments do not necessarily have a substantial body of evidence for their efficacy either—the key message is often just to use a nonopioid-based treatment.

In May 2019, the U.S. Department of Health and Human Services (HHS) released a report titled "Pain Management Best Practices" [18], which was generated by a multidisciplinary, inter agency task force assembled by the HHS. The mission of this task force was to identify gaps, inconsistencies, and new information that could potentially better inform how acute and chronic pain should be managed, especially with respect to the use of opioid analgesics as part of a pain treatment plan. The main theme with respect to the use of medications like opioids to treat chronic pain was that the decision to incorporate them into a treatment plan should be based on a solid foundation of a detailed pain-related history and physical examination, a presumptive or definitive diagnosis, and thorough understanding about the mechanisms involved in the particular type of pain diagnosis, and a risk-benefit assessment which "demonstrates that the benefits of a medication [choice] outweigh the risks" of the individual patient, their context, and individual circumstances.

This report also included an analysis and review of the impact of the 2016 CDC Guidelines and acknowledged that there were "unintended consequences" of these guidelines resulting in some cases from misinterpretation, misapplication, or both, which included forced tapering of patients on long-term opioid therapy, or even in some cases patient abandonment.

This report recommended that there should be development of diagnosis-based pain management best practices which are incorporated into medical and dental practices, and clinical health systems, with achievement of this resulting from incorporation of these practices into the "routine training of clinicians." Additionally, this report stressed that from a payer perspective, when appropriate, nonopioid-based therapies needed to be adequately covered and reimbursed, reinforcing the idea that the best approach to treating pain incorporates a multimodal approach. The report stated that regardless of the modality selected, whether it be medication, restorative therapy, interventional treatment, behavioral therapy, or complementary/integrative health-based, that **four critical topics** needed to be considered which will inform them. These four topics are **risk assessment**, **stigma**, **access to care**, and **education**.

This report acknowledged many existing gaps in pain care related to opioid therapy including (but not limited to): (1) current inconsistencies and fragment of pain care are a significant issue in healthcare today, and a "coherent policy for *all* relevant stakeholders is needed"; (2) "there has been minimal pain education in medical school and residency programs, and little guidance for PCPs on appropriate pain treatment approaches with opioids and nonopioid therapies"; (3) "education is currently inadequate for patients and clinicians regarding safe medication storage and appropriate disposal of excess medications targeted at reducing outstanding supplies of opioids that others can misuse or that children and other vulnerable members of the household can inadvertently access"; and (4) optimal naloxone use is "not widely understood" and implemented.

Unfortunately, despite the breadth of this report and its valuable recommendations in terms of bridging existing gaps, especially with respect to opioid analgesic use in both acute and chronic pain management, dissemination of this report has not been widely achieved, allowing for continued propagation of continuing lack of consensus. A familiar dilemma.

References

1. Dowell D, Haegerich TM, Chou R. CDC guideline for prescribing opioids for chronic pain – United States, 2016. MMWR Recomm Rep. 2016;65(1):1–49.
2. Benintendi A, Kosakowski S, Lagisetty P, Larochelle M, Bohnert ASB, Bazzi AR. "I felt like I had a scarlet letter": recurring experiences of structural stigma surrounding opioid tapers among patients with chronic, non-cancer pain. Drug Alcohol Depend. 2021;222:108664.
3. Katz NP, Adams EH, Chilcoat H, Colucci RD, Comer SD, Goliber P, Grudzinskas C, Jasinski D, Lande SD, Passik SD, Schnoll SH, Sellers E, Travers D, Weiss R. Challenges in the development of prescription opioid abuse-deterrent formulations. Clin J Pain. 2007;23(8):648–60.
4. The American Medical Association. Physicians' actions to help end the nation's drug-related overdose and death epidemic—and what still needs to be done. 2021, 2022, 2023. https://end-overdose-epidemic.org/. Accessed 22 June 2024.
5. Barreveld AM. As a pain specialist, I may have caused more harm by under-prescribing opioids. STAT. 2022, April 12. https://www.statnews.com/2022/04/12/underprescribing-opioids-can-also-cause-harm/. Accessed 23 June 2023.
6. Szalavitz M. What the opioid crisis took from people in pain. The New York Times. 2022, March 7.
7. Agnoli A, Xing G, Tancredi DJ, Magnan E, Jerant A, Fenton JJ. Association of dose tapering with overdose or mental health crisis among patients prescribed long-term opioids. JAMA. 2021;326(5):411–9. Erratum in: JAMA. 2022 Feb 15;327(7):688. Erratum in: JAMA. 2022 Feb 15;327(7):687.
8. Dowell D, Haegerich T, Chou R. No shortcuts to safer opioid prescribing. N Engl J Med. 2019;380(24):2285–7.
9. Haffajee RL. Prescription drug monitoring programs – friend or folly in addressing the opioid-overdose crisis? N Engl J Med. 2019;381(8):699–701.
10. U.S. Food and Drug Administration. Risk Evaluation and Mitigation Strategies (REMS). 2023, May 16. https://www.fda.gov/drugs/drug-safety-and-availability/risk-evaluation-and-mitigation-strategies-rems. Accessed 23 June 2023.
11. REMS Program Committee. Opioid analgesic REMS. https://www.opioidanalgesicrems.com/home.html. Accessed 23 June 2023.
12. Comerci G Jr, Katzman J, Duhigg D. Controlling the swing of the opioid pendulum. N Engl J Med. 2018;378(8):691–3.
13. Rieder TN. There's never just one side to the story: why America must stop swinging the opioid pendulum. Narrat Inq Bioeth. 2018;8(3):225–31.
14. Office of National Drug Control Policy, President Barack Obama, The White House. National drug control strategy. 2011. https://obamawhitehouse.archives.gov/ondcp/2011-national-drug-control-strategy. Accessed 20 June 2023.
15. Clark C. California medical board to revise dreaded death certificate project. MedPage Today. 2020, November 17.

16. Lembke A, Humphreys K, Newmark J. Weighing the risks and benefits of chronic opioid therapy. Am Fam Physician. 2016;93(12):982–90.
17. Von Korff M, Kolodny A, Deyo RA, Chou R. Long-term opioid therapy reconsidered. Ann Intern Med. 2011;155(5):325–8.
18. U.S. Department of Health and Human Services. Pain management best practices inter-agency task force report: updates, gaps, inconsistencies, and recommendations. 2019, May. Retrieved June 23, 2023. U. S. Department of Health and Human Services website: https://www.hhs.gov/ash/advisory-committees/pain/reports/index.html

Bias, Stigma, and Social Determinants of Health

8

Introduction

Pain is ubiquitous and experienced differently by individuals based on biological, cultural, and psychosocial factors. The 2003 Institute of Medicine (IOM) report *Unequal Treatment: Confronting Racial and Ethnic Disparities in Health Care* [1] concluded that racial and ethnic minorities received lower quality general health services even when variables such as insurance status, access to healthcare, health status, comorbid conditions, and socioeconomic factors were controlled for. This landmark study determined that "…bias, prejudice, and stereotyping on the part of health care providers may contribute to differences in care" [1]. This conclusion sent shockwaves through the healthcare community as it was one of the first comprehensive, nationally released reports examining racial and ethnic disparities in the United States. The 2003 report, *The Unequal Burden of Pain*, added evidence supporting the findings of the IOM report, concluding "…racial and ethnic disparities in pain perception, assessment, and treatment were found in all settings (i.e., postoperative, emergency room) and across all types of pain (i.e., acute, cancer, chronic nonmalignant, and experimental)" [2].

Health inequity (or disparity, used interchangeably in this chapter), defined in the early 1990s, refers to "differences that are not only unnecessary and avoidable, but in addition, are considered unfair and unjust" [3]. The definition of health disparity has evolved to encompass the "preventable differences in the burden of disease, injury, violence or opportunities to achieve optimal health that are experienced by socially disadvantaged populations" (Center for Disease Control [CDC]), [4]. Socially marginalized groups are described by characteristics such as race, ethnicity, gender, age, and sexual orientation—populations that have historically experienced discrimination. Marginalized populations in the United States are more prone to the negative consequences of disparities in pain assessment and treatment. Examples of disparity in pain treatment based on race, ethnicity, and gender can be found in multiple areas such as:

© The Author(s), under exclusive license to Springer Nature Switzerland AG 2024
K. L. Zacharoff, P. Migdal, *Pain, Drugs, and Ethics*,
https://doi.org/10.1007/978-3-031-63018-7_8

- Underuse of analgesia for acute pain treatment in the emergency room
- Inadequate treatment of chronic pain
- Disparity in postsurgical pain treatment
- Undertreatment of patients in sickle cell crisis
- Decreased access to prescription medications in pharmacies in low-income neighborhoods
- Gender disparity in total knee arthroplasties
- Referrals to palliative or hospice care at the end of life

The 2011 IOM report, *Relieving Pain in America* [5], acknowledged pain as a public health challenge and highlighted disparity in the "prevalence, seriousness, and adequate treatment of pain," especially in vulnerable populations. The biomedical understanding of disease processes conflicts with the subjective nature of reported pain. Often hard to see and without verifiable laboratory or radiological testing, diagnosing and adequately treating pain is challenging for a healthcare system that relies on objective findings. This lack of evidence-based decision-making may partly account for the influence that stigma, bias, and the social determinants of health (SDoH) have on the disparity reported in the treatment of, and outcomes in, patients with acute or chronic pain.

The overarching goal of the *Healthy People Report 2030* [6], published every 10 years by the Department of Health and Human Services (DHHS), is not just to eliminate health disparity but to achieve health equity and includes the reduction of adults with chronic pain affecting work and activities of daily living. Described as a moral imperative the relief of pain must include "… a cultural transformation in the way pain is viewed and treated" [5]. This shift encompasses a move away from the traditional biomedical approach toward an interdisciplinary approach that assesses pain through a biopsychosocial lens. Such an approach includes understanding how individual, clinician, and structural factors influence and perpetuate disparity in pain treatment. This chapter will focus on the underlying impact that bias, stigma, and the social determinants of health (SDoH) have on health disparities in the assessment, management, and outcomes of treatment for acute and chronic pain.

Bias and Health Disparity

Inequality in pain management has persisted in the decades following the landmark report *Unequal Treatment* [1] despite the introduction of standards of care by the Joint Commission in 2001 for organizations to improve pain care management, significant research, and considerable cost to society related to loss of productivity, poorer quality of life, and increased disability. Marginalized patient populations, including women, and adults and children of color remain vulnerable to poorer care of pain. Bias, or "the negative [or positive] evaluation of one group and its members relative to another" [7], is considered ubiquitous in the population including healthcare providers even though most healthcare professionals enter medicine with egalitarian goals [8]. Treatment decisions by healthcare professionals are more likely to be unintentionally influenced by their own judgments and implicit attitudes due to the subjective nature of pain. Implicit bias has been implicated as a contributor to the development and persistence of health disparities in pain. Unlike explicit bias, in which an individual is aware of their beliefs, implicit bias is quickly and automatically activated at an unconscious level and may influence communication and clinical decision-making in health care [9, 10].

Bias develops due to the natural categorization processes of the human brain that are needed to organize the surrounding environment to make everyday decisions rapidly and efficiently. Social categorization begins at a young age and is influenced by family, culture, media, and other lived experiences. This process leads to the overgeneralization or stereotyping of social groups without consideration of characteristics unique to the individual [11]. In the discussion of disparities in pain assessment and treatment, Tait and Chibnall [12] note, "Because pain is a subjective phenomenon that often defies objective medical assessment, it is particularly susceptible to social psychological influences, such as stereotypes." In addition, these unintentional biases are hard to root out due to a lack of recognition of one's own biases. Wang and Jeon [13] found that cognitive bias influences the belief of individuals that others, not themselves, are susceptible to social biases in everyday encounters.

Racial and Ethnic Bias and Disparity in Pain Treatment

Acute pain is a common reason for visits to the emergency department (ED) [14]. After controlling for pain severity, Singhal, Tien, and Hsai [15] compared prescribing patterns for opioid administration while in the ED and opioid prescription at the time of discharge for subjective versus objective pain, namely, abdominal pain, back pain, versus long-bone fractures, and kidney stones. All racial and ethnic minorities were less likely to receive opioid analgesia in the ED and at discharge for abdominal pain; this pattern was also found for back pain in non-Hispanic Blacks compared to non-Hispanic White patients. A recent meta-analysis added support that racial and ethnic minorities are often undertreated for pain in the acute setting [16]. This review concluded that compared to White patients, Black and Hispanic patients were less likely to receive any analgesia, including opioid medications for acute pain and that these differences were not associated with requests for different dosages of pain medications.

Reports of disparity in the treatment of chronic pain are also well documented. According to a 2011 review by Mossey [17], "African Americans are less likely than whites to receive opioid analgesics for chronic pain conditions and/or other treatments, such as referral to surgery." Morales and Yong [18] reviewed over 50 studies between 2000 and 2020 examining disparity in chronic pain treatment. This review substantiated reports that racial and ethnic disparities continue to persist in the treatment of chronic pain. Settings of disparity varied widely, including findings that minorities in nursing homes were more likely than Whites to have uncontrolled pain, Black patients prescribed opioids for chronic pain in a primary care setting reported higher levels of disability and lower quality of life measures compared to White patients and this was related to higher perceived discrimination and hopelessness, and self-reported breakthrough of pain and lower quality of life was found in minority patients with cancer-related pain [19–21].

Adding to the evidence of the persistence of disparate pain treatment are the results of a 2021 study reported in the *New England Journal of Medicine*. Morden and colleagues [22] examined patterns of opioid prescription between Blacks and Whites using a national sample of Medicare claims from 2016 to 2017 to analyze differences within 310 individual health systems. The results were startling, not only confirming unequal treatment of pain based on race but also finding biased prescribing patterns within most individual health systems. Within the same health system not only were Black patients less likely to receive an opioid prescription than White patients but when a prescription opioid was given the mean annual dosage was significantly less among Black patients. The analysis revealed bias in opioid prescribing and concluded:

> Despite the limitations in our data, it is hard to imagine that, within each of the 310 health systems that we studied, the differences in need, preferences, and opioid-associated risks among White patients and Black patients explain such substantial inequality in opioid receipt.

Bias is implicated in the persistence of racial and ethnic disparities in chronic pain assessment and treatment over decades raising questions about the efficacy of clinical practice in the pursuit of equity in the management of pain.

Disparity in the treatment of pain is described in the pediatric population. The 2015 review of National Hospital Ambulatory Medical Care Survey (NHAMCS) data of nearly one million children with known appendicitis presenting to the ED revealed that compared to White children, Black children were significantly less likely to receive any analgesia for moderate pain [23]. Use of any analgesia was comparable for treatment of severe pain, but Black children were significantly less likely to receive a prescription opioid, having an odds ratio of just 0.2 compared to White children. According to the authors "Our findings suggest that although clinicians may recognize pain equally across all racial groups, they may be reacting to the pain differently by treating black patients with nonopioid analgesia, such as ibuprofen and acetaminophen, while treating white patients with opioid analgesia for similar pain." The subjective reporting of abdominal pain associated with appendicitis raises concern that unconscious, implicit biases influence physician treatment decisions in pain management.

Similarly, a 2021 retrospective study of over 13,000 children evaluated in the ED at Boston Children's Hospital for either a limb fracture or suspected appendicitis revealed racial and ethnic disparity in pain management of these conditions. The results suggest, "The differences most likely represent true racial inequities with an under prescription of opioids for Back Non-Hispanic (NH) and Hispanic children" [24]. Notably, despite increased pain severity in non-White patients at initial evaluation, opioid medication was prescribed less for both Black NH and Hispanic children than NH White children raising concern that implicit biases influence treatment decisions in the acute setting.

Factors Associated with Bias in the Treatment of Pain

How does bias influence treatment decisions and outcomes for pain management? Examining the causes of disparate pain outcomes helps guide solutions to alleviate the inequitable treatment of pain. The negative consequences of bias in pain assessment have been attributed to several factors. Cognitive stressors in the working environment that arise in medicine—working under time pressure, fatigue, clinical uncertainty, overcrowded EDs, and higher patient load—are conditions associated with increased reliance on implicit, unconscious biases [25–27]. Consequences of stereotyping and biases against racial and ethnic minority patients have been shown to negatively affect communication, trust, and decision-making among healthcare professionals [9, 28].

Sabin and Greenwald [29] used the implicit association test (IAT) to study the impact of race on treatment recommendations in pediatricians. Developed in the 1990s, the IAT is a computer-based test involving the rapid categorization of concepts to measure implicit attitudes about characteristics such as race or gender. These investigators administered three different IATs to a group of pediatricians—a Race IAT, Race-Medical Compliance IAT, and Race-Quality of Care IAT—to investigate possible associations with differences in recommendations of care after viewing pediatric clinical vignettes that varied only by the race of the patient, e.g., African American, or White. Higher measurements of pro-White implicit bias were significantly associated with the likelihood of recommending a prescription narcotic post-surgery in the case of pain management for a 14-year-old White male patient than for a Black child in the same vignette.

The accurate perception of pain influences clinical decision-making. Lack of empathy and perspective-taking by the provider toward the patient has the potential to lead to inadequate treatment of pain [30, 31]. Physician empathy may be thought of as "…the socio-emotional competence of a physician to be able to understand the patient's situation, perspective, and feelings, to communicate that understanding and check its accuracy, and to act on that understanding with the patient in a helpful (therapeutic) way" [32]. Studying the degree of empathy elicited, researchers from Italy demonstrated decreased responses to pain by White respondents when viewing African versus White subjects and that this decreased empathic response was associated with increased implicit race bias [33]. Conversely, other studies have demonstrated a positive effect of increased clinician empathy on improved patient outcomes, increased information sharing, and improved quality of life [32–34].

Drwecki and colleagues [30] examined the influence of empathy and perspective-taking on disparity in pain treatment. Perspective-taking or understanding an individual's circumstances from another point of view has been shown to positively impact patient satisfaction in a clinical setting [35]. Nurses watched videos of an examination of a patient with shoulder pain varying only by patient race, Black or

White. The control group was instructed to make the "best, most accurate treatment decisions for each patient." The perspective-taking participants had further instruction—"attempt to imagine how each of your patients feels while you are examining them"—and this perspective-taking intervention was reinforced before and after viewing the video, with a statement such as, "spend a moment imagining how your patient feels about his or her pain and how this pain is affecting their life." A 65% reduction in treatment bias toward Blacks was found in the perspective-taking group compared to the control group.

Supporting the positive role of empathy on outcomes in patients with chronic pain, recent research examined the perception of physician empathy by chronic pain patients. This study showed greater improvement in average pain intensity and health-related quality-of-life measures as patient's perception of physician empathy increased leading the authors to suggest that "Physicians' empathy may therefore be a suitable, yet relatively unexplored, target for intervention" to decrease the disparity in pain treatment outcomes [36].

Studies have found that both the general population and healthcare professionals believe that Blacks feel less pain than Whites [37, 38]. Researchers at the University of Virginia [39] sought to explicate the mechanism that underlies inaccurate perceptions and treatment recommendations of pain based on race by examining belief in biological differences between Blacks and Whites by medical students and residents. At least one false belief, such as Black people have thicker skin than Whites or that Blacks' nerve endings are less sensitive than Whites' were believed by 50% of the participants. These false beliefs were associated with inaccurate pain perception in Blacks and inadequate treatment recommendations. False biological beliefs leading to differences in pain perception and treatment between Blacks and Whites may contribute to the persistence of these disparities.

Gender Bias and Disparity in Pain Treatment

Undertreatment of pain in women has long been described with evidence supporting gender bias [40]. Research suggests that women have a higher likelihood of painful conditions such as musculoskeletal pain, fibromyalgia, migraine, and abdominal pain that may lead to greater disability than in men [41, 42]. The prevalence of painful conditions in women is generally considered multifactorial related to biological, hormonal, cultural, and societal expectations that underlie gender stereotypes [41]. Even though women are more likely to perceive and discuss their pain with healthcare providers, they are also less likely to be taken seriously, have their pain attributed to psychosocial etiologies, and receive treatment with anxiolytics or antidepressants rather than pain medications [40].

In a study examining the treatment of acute abdominal pain in an urban ED, women compared to men had longer wait times for treatment and were 13% to15% less likely to receive an opioid analgesic [43]. Examination of emergency medical services (EMS) found differences in receipt of evidence-based recommended treatments, lower use of sirens and lights during transport, and a lower likelihood of receiving out-of-hospital resuscitation for women with chest pain [44]. NHAMCS data from 2014 to 2018 revealed that women presenting to the ED with chest pain were less likely to be triaged as an emergency and waited longer for evaluation than men [45].

A 2018 literature review by Samulowitz and colleagues [46], *"Brave Men and Emotional Women"* examining various causes of pain, such as back pain, musculoskeletal pain, fibromyalgia syndrome and arthritis discusses evidence implicating gender bias in pain assessment. These gendered beliefs included differences in how men and women experience pain, cope with pain, strive (women) to be believed about their pain, and experience bias in pain management. Over a broad range of settings, including researchers, men experiencing pain, and healthcare providers, men were considered more stoic and autonomous and less likely to seek medical care or discuss pain. Conversely, women were described as more sensitive to and willing to discuss pain symptoms. Pain in women was more likely to be viewed as "hysterical, emotional, complaining, … fabricating the pain, as if it is all in her head" [46]. Clinicians had a harder time believing their patients for "medically inexplicable pain," pain that was described as purely subjective such as fibromyalgia. One study reported that physicians found these patients more frustrating to work with and questioned if the patient was responsible for their pain. This review confirmed what was reported by Hoffmann and Tarzian [40] over two decades ago: gender stereotypes influence the treatment of women with pain conditions and help to explain why women are less likely to be prescribed pain medications and more likely to be referred to a mental health specialist than men.

In conclusion, the etiology of bias and its resulting disparity in pain treatment is multifold. Awareness of the clinical impact of bias is necessary to mitigate its negative effects to close the gap in the disparity of pain treatment. Research repeatedly demonstrates that pain may be underestimated and inadequately treated based on factors such as race, ethnicity, and gender. Studies have shed light about underlying factors that affect how bias impacts the assessment of pain and treatment decisions. Further investigation is still necessary, as Morales and Yong [18] simply state "A clear understanding of disparities within the treatment of chronic [and acute] pain is essential to creating and implementing effective interventions for vulnerable populations." Reliance on stereotypes, lack of empathy toward certain populations, false beliefs, and one's working environment have been shown to impact biased responses and lead to disparity in the care of patients with pain. These detrimental effects on clinical decision-making are a reminder of the importance of continued education about the role bias in the assessment and treatment of pain:

> Racial and ethnic disparities in pain treatment are not intentional misdeeds: health care providers do not decide that some groups deserve pain relief while others should suffer. Instead, inequities are the product of complex influences, including implicit biases that care providers don't even know they have [47].

Awareness of the impact of bias, educational initiatives for clinicians, institutional reimagining regarding the delivery of care for pain management, and policy change are important areas to examine to enable the necessary changes to achieve equity in the treatment of people seeking medical care for pain.

Stigma

Stigma perpetuates disparity and acts as a roadblock to the achievement of well-being for the millions of people experiencing pain, require opioids to relieve pain, or have a substance use disorder (SUD). Stigma, identified as a mark of shame [48] devalues the individual and creates a milieu ripe for discrimination. The consequences of stigma in healthcare occur "when a label associated with a negative stereotype is attached to a characteristic (race, disease) causing people with this characteristic to be seen as separate from and lower in status than others and thus, as legitimate targets of discrimination" [49]. The consequences of this "us versus other" stereotyping support the conclusion that stigma is a fundamental cause of health inequities [50].

Feelings of stigma have been reported by patients who have met resistance to social interactions, including in healthcare. "I felt very stigmatized. I feel like I'm wearing a scarlet letter," "I hate that I am being treated like a drug abuser when I am just trying to make my life more manageable…Not everyone who needs pain relief is an abuser," "I was accused of drug seeking, belittled for having a low pain threshold… and dismissed as a patient" [51, 52]. These are among a sample of perspectives from patients treated for chronic pain with opioids and give credence to how stigma may negatively impact healthcare for these patients.

The cascading effects of stigma can be organized into three domains: first, the patient or intrapersonal level; second, the clinician or interpersonal level; and finally, the societal level manifesting in structural stigma. When these different levels of stigma act during a patient encounter involving the subjective evaluation of pain, health outcomes suffer. These intersecting dimensions of stigma lead to a variety of consequences such as treatment avoidance by patients, negative attitudes of providers of care, negative attitudes toward the providers of care, lack of access to care, poorer quality of care, and institutional policies that contribute to an environment of mistrust, and inadvertently further disenfranchise persons with pain [52–54].

There are two types of intrapersonal stigma: anticipated and internalized. Anticipated stigma may be thought of as the expectation of being rejected because of one's awareness of negative attitudes surrounding their stigmatized condition [55]. Internalized stigma is defined as the acceptance of the negative stereotypes associated with pain; each is correlated with poorer patient outcomes [55, 56]. A 2014 survey of patients with chronic pain revealed that 38% experienced internalized stigma which was inversely correlated to self-esteem and self-efficacy [56]. A statement by a patient with chronic pain treated with opioid medication—"I'm made to feel like a criminal"—provides an example of how intrapersonal stigma forms [52]. The impacts are wide-ranging, including increased isolation and invalidation of their experience of pain.

Slade and colleagues [57] interviewed patients with nonspecific chronic low back pain, and concluded that "the ramifications of stigma and discrimination are enduring, potentially disabling and appear to interfere with care-seeking, rehabilitation participation, and potentially, rehabilitation outcomes." The increased psychological effects of intrapersonal stigma, whether anticipated or internalized, contribute to feelings of delegitimization, shame, and decreased participation in health care. The coexistence or development of comorbid conditions, such as depression or anxiety, and the possibility of seeking illicit drugs for pain relief results in worse health outcomes in patients with pain or persons with SUD [52].

Healthcare professionals also may perpetuate stigma and negatively influence health outcomes for their patients with chronic pain. This interpersonal stigma may be described in terms of the effects of enacted stigma and public stigma. Negative stereotypes associated with chronic pain patients underlie public stigma. Enacted stigma refers to the behavioral manifestations of public stigma "that lead to delivery of suboptimal care and undermine access to treatment and harm reduction services" [55]. Studies evaluating stigma of chronic pain patients prescribed opioids suggest varying beliefs about the negative assumptions of these patients. These stigmatizing attitudes include disbelief due to the lack of objective, biomedical findings related to the complaint of pain and believing that opioid therapy is not an effective treatment. Additionally, there may be concern about associated SUD or medication diversion in patients prescribed opioids for chronic pain [58].

Compounding stigma for patients with chronic pain is the difficulty patients have in finding physicians willing to treat them. A penalty is observed for patients prescribed opioids for chronic pain seeking care from a new PCP. As one of the investigators of these studies, Pooja Lagisetty, states, "Even if you think that someone is using opioids for a reason other than pain, or that long-term opioids are not an effective strategy, those are exactly the patients we in primary care should be seeing" [59]. Ample research supports that some physicians hold stigmatizing attitudes toward patients with chronic pain especially if treated with opioids. This amplifies disparity and leads to further internalization of stigma, including feelings of shame, lower self-esteem, isolation, and treatment avoidance as well as difficulty finding a treating physician, general feelings of distrust in the healthcare system, and lower quality of care [60].

Lagisetty and colleagues [61] examined the willingness of primary care clinics to accept new patients with a history of chronic pain prescribed opioids. Just over 40% of the clinics surveyed refused new patients regardless of insurance type. Lagisetty and others [60] then designed a "secret shopper" survey to evaluate the acceptance by primary care physicians (PCP) of chronic pain patients treated with opioids in nine states providing two scenarios by callers posing as new patients. The scenarios differed in the explanation of seeking a new practice; the premise of needing a new patient appointment in scenario one was due to their previous physician retiring and in scenario two was due to their physician stopping their prescription of opioid medication without explanation. A large percentage of offices (40%) would not prescribe opioids in either case scenario. Twenty-five percent of the clinics responded differently to the scenarios—offices were more likely to continue to prescribe an opioid if the previous physician retired versus stopped prescribing without explanation.

The shortage of primary care physicians and pain specialists to treat the millions of patients with pain may be affected by the concept of courtesy stigma, or "the process through which one's identity is tainted by virtue of their association with the directly stigmatized individual" [62]. As described by the DHHS, this kind of stigma potentially affects some clinicians treating patients with pain, especially when prescription opioids are needed. Concern about how one's professional reputation may be affected by this type of stigma and fear of scrutiny from state regulatory boards and the Drug Enforcement Administration (DEA) may influence a clinician's willingness to treat patients with pain (HHS Fact Sheet) [63].

Finally, structural stigma impedes treatment of chronic pain patients. Public and enacted stigma may develop into structural stigma when stigma becomes accepted and incorporated into culture, institutions, and legal systems. An environment of mistrust and inadequate treatment may develop due to external forces that limit needed resources and empathic and compassionate care to a large group of patients [55].

Structural stigma was inadvertently heightened in 2016 when the CDC released a report providing recommendations for opioid prescribing in response to the burgeoning opioid crisis and the increasing number of deaths due to drug overdoses [64]. Though the intent was in response to the recognition of the worsening opioid crisis, the consequences led to devastating outcomes for the many patients prescribed opioids that were used successfully in the treatment of chronic pain without evidence of negative consequences of addiction. Meant to be guidelines for opioid prescribing that specifically excluded patients in active cancer treatment, palliative care, or end-of-life care, these guidelines were codified into law by many states or considered mandates regarding opioid prescribing for all patients. Several state legislatures passed laws limiting the amount of medication that could be prescribed. By 2018 over 30 states had laws regulating opioid prescriptions [65]. Recent studies conclude that there has been an increase in overdose, suicide, or hospitalizations due to mental illness after opioid taper or discontinuation [66, 67].

The CDC updated the clinical practice guidelines in response to the observed detrimental effects of the 2016 recommendations. These original guidelines led to institutional policies regulating the dosage, number of prescriptions, and monitoring of patients treated with opioids for chronic pain. Finding a physician willing to treat chronic pain with opioids even at the end of life became increasingly difficult during this time and left patients suffering and feeling abandoned by the health care system. The first case of its type, Slone versus Commonwealth Pain Associates, PLLC was recently decided in favor of the family of a man on chronic opioid treatment for pain after the patient's prescription pain medication was involuntarily and unknowingly decreased. The office refused to provide additional pain medication until a subsequent follow-up 6 days later. After multiple attempts to get a prescription for the few days until the appointment, the patient Brent Slone, committed suicide. This multimillion dollar award is the first to side against physicians for an involuntary opioid taper [68].

The striking consequences of stigma on intrapersonal, interpersonal, and structural levels have led to distrust in the system of healthcare, healthcare provider concerns about treating patients with chronic pain, especially if the patient requires opioids, and policies that are not flexible enough to regard patients with chronic pain as individuals with different needs. Given the complex multilevel causes creating a medical environment of stigma, solutions need to be considered that address each of these areas.

Being mindful about and changing stigmatizing language associated with chronic pain and SUD may lessen the impact of stigma. An examination of stigmatizing language in electronic health records (EHR) noted three areas of stigmatizing language use based on diagnosis including patients diagnosed with SUD and patients with chronic pain (the third was diabetes). Stigmatizing language was more likely in descriptors of non-Hispanic Blacks than non-Hispanic White patients. Stigmatizing descriptors in the EHR of patients with SUD or chronic pain included, "Avoid narcotics given the history of abuse," "Concern for secondary gain given narcotic seeking behavior," and "Questionable if hyperalgesia or drug seeking behavior" [69]. Removing blame and increasing empathy through modifying the language associated with substance use may decrease stigma. For example, referring to a patient as a person with a substance use disorder versus a substance abuser was found to have fewer negative connotations [70]. The same is true for decreasing the use of stigmatizing language on a structural level such as consideration of changing the name of a leading federal organization, *National Institute of Drug Abuse,* to create a less stigmatizing environment for patients with chronic pain or SUD.

As noted above, the CDC has updated the guidelines for opioid prescribing, and this may help decrease the stigma associated with using this class of medication for the treatment of pain and have positive effects on decreasing the existing structural stigma associated with pain management. Awareness and education may begin to lessen interpersonal stigma and the resulting negative effects on patient care, which have left people in pain suffering, or, worse, feeling abandoned by the clinicians that are meant to provide care. Medical education is still woefully inadequate with most medical schools in the United States having no mandatory curricula on pain [71]. Understanding stigma and staying informed about best practices, and the benefit of multimodal treatments, can be achieved through continuing education requirements. Educational benefits may also include increased empathy and compassion in the care of patients by enhancing understanding of how stigma affects pain treatment.

Finally, creating a less stigmatizing environment in healthcare may help alleviate the negative intrapersonal stigma by decreasing the internalized stigma felt by these patients. Education, counseling, and reflective writing had positive results in other groups of stigmatized and vulnerable patients, for example, people living with HIV/AIDS [49]. Accepting and understanding patients' pain instead of blaming creates an environment of trust and better communication between the patient and health care provider. The effect of improved self-efficacy and confidence will benefit all involved and increase equity in the treatment of pain.

Social Determinants of Health

Appreciation of the influence of SDoH has gained prominence over the last several decades in unpacking the root causes of health disparity, including for the treatment of pain. These factors influence health, health-related behavior, and well-being. The SDoH are defined as "the conditions in the environments where people are born, live, learn, work, play, worship, and age that affect a wide range of health, functioning, and quality-of-life outcomes and risks" [6]. These conditions are shaped by a wider set of forces: economics, social policies, and politics (World Health Organization [WHO]) [72].

The SDoH are generally grouped into five domains: (1) economic stability, (2) education access and quality, (3) neighborhood and built environment, (4) social and community context, and (5) health care access and quality [6]. The COVID-19 pandemic turned national attention to the interpersonal and structural effects of racism (not the social construct of race) as a factor affecting the SDoH as significant inequality in morbidity and mortality due to COVID-19 in populations of color was reported [73]. As the pandemic gripped the country, limitations of chronic pain services led to increased isolation and psychosocial consequences in persons with chronic pain [74].

The import of the SDoH is considerable especially since overall health behaviors, social and economic factors such as income level, access to quality education, and neighborhood characteristics, e.g., availability of transportation, green spaces, and affordable healthy food options, have a greater impact on well-being than health care services alone [75]. Approximately 20% of health is determined to be modifiable through medical care; the other SDoH domains influence the larger proportion of factors that affect health and well-being [76]. The groundbreaking research by Sir Michael Marmot beginning in the 1960s led to the current understanding that a social gradient of health exists, or, in other words, there is no absolute cutoff of income or education above which all people achieve the same level of health. A continuing inverse relationship is found: the lower one's socioeconomic status (SES) the higher likelihood of illness and decreased life expectancy [77].

Sociodemographic factors lead to a healthcare system that hinders health equity achievement in emergency and outpatient settings for patients presenting with pain. Pain is a common reason for ED visits and outpatient consultations and social determinants influence the assessment and management of pain conditions. Higher levels of poverty and lower levels of education are associated with worse outcomes in the treatment of acute and chronic pain. Neighborhood characteristics and rurality influence the availability of primary care providers and pain management specialists adding to the difficulty of receiving adequate care for pain [5]. Awareness of the influence of SDoH on outcomes related to pain care is thus a crucial aspect of improving quality of life, decreasing healthcare costs, and lessening health disparity in the care of pain conditions.

Joynt and colleagues [78] examined the impact of neighborhood socioeconomic status (SES) and race on the likelihood of receiving an opioid prescription for moderate to severe pain. Using data from the NHAMCS, this group examined over

50,000 visits to EDs from different regions of the United States. Patients with lower SES, patients living in areas with higher rates of poverty and lower educational achievement, were less likely to receive prescribed opioids for moderate to severe pain. This study also confirmed that regardless of SES, opioids were less often prescribed for Black and Hispanic patients compared to White patients. These findings support the association between race, ethnicity, poverty, and pain management reported in the 2011 IOM Report: *Relieving Pain in America* [5].

Outpatient treatment of patients with chronic pain follows a similar pattern found in the ED and links SDoH to disparate outcomes. Musculoskeletal pain, such as chronic back pain, and osteoarthritis places a significant burden on healthcare, and leads to disability in this population [79]. A literature review examining disparity in the treatment of chronic pain by Morales and Yong [18] concluded that "these studies support the hypothesis that a patient's sociodemographic profile influences the treatment of their chronic pain." For example, a review of the impact of SDoH on outcomes in patients with lower back pain found that lower socioeconomic status and educational level have the strongest association with the prevalence and severity of chronic lower back pain [79].

Surgical treatment of joint dysfunction may be recommended to improve function and pain. Yet, despite, for instance, the similar prevalence of joint dysfunction between Black and White patients, and increased reporting of disparity over the last several decades, inequity in joint replacement surgery continues [80]. Income and education affected surgical outcomes for the treatment of low back pain: lower income and educational levels were associated with poorer outcomes after surgery, described as postoperative disability and pain [81].

A comprehensive study reviewing regional referral patterns by Thirukumaran and colleagues [82] revealed that disparities have persisted or increased between 2009 and 2017 for total knee replacement and total hip replacement, respectively, based on SES and race. Variables analyzed included race, Black or White, and SES, using Medicare-only beneficiaries versus Medicare/Medicaid eligible (dual-eligibility beneficiaries) as a proxy for SES. Black and White dual-eligibility beneficiaries had lower surgical rates for both knee and hip replacement than Medicare-only beneficiaries. Within each socioeconomic group Blacks consistently had fewer joint replacements than their White counterparts. Regional referral patterns revealed geographic disparity: areas that had a higher proportion of Black or dual-eligible beneficiaries had significantly lower rates of joint replacement surgeries. Geographic factors leading to disparity have been attributed to the lack of resources in poor and/or highly segregated neighborhoods affecting access to healthcare services [83]. As the authors state, "Efforts to improve equity must identify and address both racial and socioeconomic barriers and focus on regions with high concentrations of disadvantaged beneficiaries."

The association between SDoH and total cost of care and lengths of hospital stays after total knee arthroplasty (TKA) was examined by Delanois and colleagues [84]. Longer lengths of stay were associated with divorced marital status and neighborhoods with a greater density of tobacco stores, a proxy used for social deprivation. Living in food deserts and a greater number of tobacco stores were significantly associated with an increased total cost of care. These authors were among the first to examine the influence of SDoH and outcomes of TKA on length of stays and healthcare costs and concluded, "In order to determine which SDOH have the greatest impact on TKA, future studies must start including the SDOH into models that predict the needs of patients at the time of admission to the hospital." Policies that address the SDoH have the potential benefits of not only improving the quality of life for people in pain but also lowering overall healthcare costs.

The SDoH have been shown to influence disparity in the assessment and management of pain. Beyond structural and individual factors such as access to adequate care, health behaviors, and patient preferences, other factors have recently been examined to explain the link between SDoH and poorer pain treatment. Asking, "Why do low-SES individuals receive substandard pain care?" Summers and colleagues [85] examined if biases exist and influence pain perception based on SES. This group designed experiments to test the hypothesis that poorer people are perceived to have less sensitivity to pain and are consequently believed to need less treatment for pain. The results supported the conclusion that lower-SES individuals are perceived as feeling less pain by both lay people and medical professionals based on the assumption that lower SES individuals "have been toughened up by prior life hardships." Most strikingly, these false beliefs and stereotypes by medical professionals led to inadequate pain treatment recommendations.

The National Center for Education Statistics estimates that 43 million adults in the United States have low literacy skills (NCES, 2019). This data suggests that this often-overlooked factor needs to be considered in treatment recommendations for patients with pain. Described as "… the personal characteristics and social resources needed for people and communities to access, understand, appraise, and use information and services to make decisions about health," health literacy impacts the effectiveness of treatment [86]. The concern is that patients with lower health literacy may not have adequate comprehension of the multimodal treatment options for the management of chronic pain.

Greater intensity of pain and lower physical functioning were associated with lower levels of health literacy for patients studied in the United Kingdom with musculoskeletal pain related to self-management recommendations over a 6-month period [86]. Controlling for confounding variables (anxiety, depression, age, gender, income, and education), Rogers and colleagues [87] found that lower health literacy was inversely associated with the likelihood of opioid misuse, worse pain intensity, and pain disability. The worse experience of pain related to lower health literacy contributes to the disparity observed in the prevalence, severity, and treatment outcomes in patients with chronic pain. These investigators suggest that further clinical research is needed to assess useful interventions for patients with chronic pain and low health literacy.

Given the diverse factors leading to inequity in pain management associated with the SDoH, remedying the disparity requires a multifocal approach. Maly and Vallerand [88] summarize the necessary steps to decrease disparity associated with chronic pain due to the social determinants of health:

> To improve the burden of chronic pain requires a multifactorial assessment that considers neighborhood risk factors, emphasis on environmental stressors, limitations to support

networks, barriers to physical activity, and access to primary care providers with whom communication is open and without bias.

Understanding, assessing, and acting on the individual, clinical, and structural factors that maintain the negative impact of SDoH is required to diminish the inequity associated with the burden that these determinants have on treatment decisions and treatment effectiveness for patients with pain.

Conclusion: Treatment of Pain—Ethical Issues

Ethics provides the grounding to do what is moral, by providing a scaffolding to determine what is right, what is wrong, and what is just or unjust. What are the ethics of care for persons in acute or chronic pain; what is the responsibility of institutions, healthcare systems, and healthcare professionals to combat the negative intrusion of bias and stigma on care? How can we address the enormity of the impact that social determinants have on health, such as SES, education, and neighborhood, on the disparate treatment of pain?

The subjective nature of pain assessment shifts the evaluation of and treatment decisions for pain toward uncertainty where the effects of bias and stigma influence decision making in ways both known and unknown. This permeates into all the multiple levels that impact care: intrapersonal, interpersonal, institutional, and cultural. Yet this subjective nature of pain assessment most alarmingly leaves patients suffering and because of bias, stigma, and social determinants of health some patients are left to suffer more than others.

Returning to the definition of health inequality described in the beginning of this chapter, "differences that are not only unnecessary and avoidable, but in addition, are considered unfair and unjust," achieving justice is both crucial and ethical to tackle the disparity in pain care due to bias, stigma, and the social determinants. Mathur and colleagues [89] discuss the mechanisms of injustice in the management of pain and conclude, "…observable disparities in pain outcomes or individual pain processes are the products of—and therefore cannot be disambiguated from – cultural, structural, and interpersonal injustice." The conclusion follows:

> Centering research and discussions about pain disparities within an injustice perspective illuminates the need for collective action to actualize justice—to be intolerant of and oppose cultural beliefs that perpetuate injustice in pain treatment, to work for societal change to end structural injustice, and to eliminate disparities in pain [89].

Seeing the patient as an individual unencumbered by stereotypes, bias, and stigma is a lofty goal. Prioritizing justice integrates the necessary upstream and downstream solutions to achieve the goal of equity in the care of patients with pain.

References

1. Smedley BD, Stith AY, Nelson AR, editors. Institute of Medicine (US) committee on under-standing and eliminating racial and ethnic disparities in health care. Unequal treatment: con-fronting racial and ethnic disparities in health care. Washington, DC: National Academies Press; 2003.
2. Green CR, Anderson KO, Baker TA, Campbell LC, Decker S, Fillingim RB, Kalauokalani DA, Lasch KE, Myers C, Tait RC, Todd KH, Vallerand AH. The unequal burden of pain: confront-ing racial and ethnic disparities in pain. Pain Med. 2003;4(3):277–94.
3. Whitehead M. The concepts and principles of equity and health. Int J Health Serv. 1992;22(3):429–45.
4. Centers for Disease Control and Prevention (2017). Alzheimer's disease and healthy aging: Health disparities. Retrieved from: https://www.cdc.gov/aging/disparities/index.htm.
5. Institute of Medicine (US) Committee on Advancing Pain Research, Care, and Education. Relieving pain in America: a blueprint for transforming prevention, care, education, and research. Washington, DC: National Academies Press; 2011.
6. The Office of Disease Prevention and Health Promotion, Office of the Assistant Secretary for Health, Office of the Secretary, U.S. Department of Health and Human Services. Healthy people. 2030. https://health.gov/healthypeople. Accessed 23 June 2023.
7. Blair IV, Steiner JF, Havranek EP. Unconscious (implicit) bias and health disparities: where do we go from here? Perm J. 2011;15(2):71–8.
8. FitzGerald C, Hurst S. Implicit bias in healthcare professionals: a systematic review. BMC Med Ethics. 2017;18:19.
9. Cooper LA, Roter DL, Carson KA, Beach MC, Sabin JA, Greenwald AG, Inui TS. The associ-ations of clinicians' implicit attitudes about race with medical visit communication and patient ratings of interpersonal care. Am J Public Health. 2012;102(5):979–87.
10. Daugherty JC, Puente AE, Fasfous AF, Hidalgo-Ruzzante N, Pérez-Garcia M. Diagnostic mis-takes of culturally diverse individuals when using North American neuropsychological tests. Appl Neuropsychol Adult. 2017;24(1):16–22.
11. Liberman Z, Woodward AL, Kinzler KD. The origins of social categorization. Trends Cogn Sci. 2017;21(7):556–68.
12. Tait RC, Chibnall JT. Racial/ethnic disparities in the assessment and treatment of pain: psycho-social perspectives. Am Psychol. 2014;69(2):131–41.
13. Wang Q, Jeon HJ. Bias in bias recognition: people view others but not themselves as biased by preexisting beliefs and social stigmas. PLoS One. 2020;15(10):e0240232.
14. Todd KH, Ducharme J, Choiniere M, Crandall CS, Fosnocht DE, Homel P, Tanabe P, PEMI Study Group. Pain in the emergency department: results of the pain and emergency medicine initiative (PEMI) multicenter study. J Pain. 2007;8(6):460–6.
15. Singhal A, Tien YY, Hsia RY. Racial-ethnic disparities in opioid prescriptions at emergency department visits for conditions commonly associated with prescription drug abuse. PLoS One. 2016;11(8):e0159224.
16. Lee P, Le Saux M, Siegel R, Goyal M, Chen C, Ma Y, Meltzer AC. Racial and ethnic disparities in the management of acute pain in US emergency departments: meta-analysis and systematic review. Am J Emerg Med. 2019;37(9):1770–7.
17. Mossey JM. Defining racial and ethnic disparities in pain management. Clin Orthop Relat Res. 2011;469(7):1859–70.
18. Morales ME, Yong RJ. Racial and ethnic disparities in the treatment of chronic pain. Pain Med. 2021;22(1):75–90.
19. Hunnicutt JN, Ulbricht CM, Tjia J, Lapane KL. Pain and pharmacologic pain management in long-stay nursing home residents. Pain. 2017;158(6):1091–9.
20. Ezenwa MO, Fleming MF. Racial disparities in pain management in primary care. J Health Dispar Res Pract. 2012;5(3):12–26.
21. Green CR, Montague L, Hart-Johnson TA. Consistent and breakthrough pain in diverse advanced cancer patients: a longitudinal examination. J Pain Symptom Manag. 2009;37(5):831–47.

22. Morden NE, Chyn D, Wood A, Meara E. Racial inequality in prescription opioid receipt – role of individual health systems. N Engl J Med. 2021;385(4):342–51.

23. Goyal MK, Kuppermann N, Cleary SD, Teach SJ, Chamberlain JM. Racial disparities in pain management of children with appendicitis in emergency departments. JAMA Pediatr. 2015;169(11):996–1002.

24. Guedj R, Marini M, Kossowsky J, Berde CB, Kimia AA, Fleegler EW. Racial and ethnic disparities in pain management of children with limb fractures or suspected appendicitis: a retrospective cross-sectional study. Front Pediatr. 2021;9:652854.

25. Stepanikova I. Racial-ethnic biases, time pressure, and medical decisions. J Health Soc Behav. 2012;53(3):329–43.

26. Tait RC, Chibnall JT, Kalauokalani D. Provider judgments of patients in pain: seeking symptom certainty. Pain Med. 2009;10(1):11–34.

27. Johnson TJ, Hickey RW, Switzer GE, Miller E, Winger DG, Nguyen M, Saladino RA, Hausmann LR. The impact of cognitive stressors in the emergency department on physician implicit racial bias. Acad Emerg Med. 2016;23(3):297–305.

28. The Joint Commission. Implicit bias in health care. Quick Safety. Issue 23. 2016, April.

29. Sabin JA, Greenwald AG. The influence of implicit bias on treatment recommendations for 4 common pediatric conditions: pain, urinary tract infection, attention deficit hyperactivity disorder, and asthma. Am J Public Health. 2012;102(5):988–95.

30. Drwecki BB, Moore CF, Ward SE, Prkachin KM. Reducing racial disparities in pain treatment: the role of empathy and perspective-taking. Pain. 2011;152(5):1001–6.

31. Penner LA, Dovidio JF, West TV, Gaertner SL, Albrecht TL, Dailey RK, Markova T. Aversive racism and medical interactions with black patients: a field study. J Exp Soc Psychol. 2010;46(2):436–40.

32. Neumann M, Wirtz M, Bollschweiler E, Mercer SW, Warm M, Wolf J, Pfaff H. Determinants and patient-reported long-term outcomes of physician empathy in oncology: a structural equation modelling approach. Patient Educ Couns. 2007;69(1–3):63–75.

33. Forgiarini M, Gallucci M, Maravita A. Racism and the empathy for pain on our skin. Front Psychol. 2011;2:108.

34. Hojat M, Louis DZ, Markham FW, Wender R, Rabinowitz C, Gonnella JS. Physicians' empathy and clinical outcomes for diabetic patients. Acad Med. 2011;86(3):359–64.

35. Blatt B, LeLaucheur SF, Galinsky AD, Simmens SJ, Greenberg L. Does perspective-takiing increase patient satisfaction in medical encounters? Academic Medicine. 2010;85(9):1445–1452.

36. Cánovas L, Carrascosa AJ, García M, Fernández M, Calvo A, Monsalve V, Soriano JF, Empathy Study Group. Impact of empathy in the patient-doctor relationship on chronic pain relief and quality of life: a prospective study in Spanish pain clinics. Pain Med. 2018;19(7):1304–14.

37. Anderson KO, Mendoza TR, Valero V, Richman SP, Russell C, Hurley J, DeLeon C, Washington P, Palos G, Payne R, Cleeland CS. Minority cancer patients and their providers: pain management attitudes and practice. Cancer. 2000;88(8):1929–38.

38. Trawalter S, Hoffman KM, Waytz A. Racial bias in perceptions of others' pain. PLoS One. 2012;7(11):e48546.

39. Hoffman KM, Trawalter S, Axt JR, Oliver MN. Racial bias in pain assessment and treatment recommendations, and false beliefs about biological differences between blacks and whites. Proc Natl Acad Sci USA. 2016;113(16):4296–301.

40. Hoffmann DE, Tarzian AJ. The girl who cried pain: a bias against women in the treatment of pain. J Law Med Ethics. 2001;29(1):13–27.

41. Doshi TL, Bicket MC. Why aren't there more female pain medicine physicians? Reg Anesth Pain Med. 2018;43(5):516–20.

42. Bartley EJ, Fillingim RB. Sex differences in pain: a brief review of clinical and experimental findings. Br J Anaesth. 2013;111(1):52–8.

43. Chen EH, Shofer FS, Dean AJ, Hollander JE, Baxt WG, Robey JL, Sease KL, Mills AM. Gender disparity in analgesic treatment of emergency department patients with acute abdominal pain. Acad Emerg Med. 2008;15(5):414–8.

44. Lewis JF, Zeger SL, Li X, Mann NC, Newgard CD, Haynes S, Wood SF, Dai M, Simon AE, McCarthy ML. Gender differences in the quality of EMS care nationwide for chest pain and out-of-hospital cardiac arrest. Womens Health Issues. 2019;29(2):116–24.
45. Banco D, Chang J, Talmor N, Wadhera P, Mukhopadhyay A, Lu X, Dong S, Lu Y, Betensky RA, Blecker S, Safdar B, Reynolds HR. Sex and race differences in the evaluation and treatment of young adults presenting to the emergency department with chest pain. J Am Heart Assoc. 2022;11(10):e024199.
46. Samulowitz A, Gremyr I, Eriksson E, Hensing G. "Brave men" and "emotional women": a theory-guided literature review on gender bias in health care and gendered norms towards patients with chronic pain. Pain Res Manag. 2018;2018:6358624.
47. Sabin JA. How we fail black patients in pain. American Association of Medical Colleges. 2020, January 6. https://www.aamc.org/news/how-we-fail-black-patients-pain. Accessed 23 June 2023.
48. Scher M. Stigma—the mark of shame. The Carter Center. 2006, April 30. https://www.carter-center.org/news/documents/doc2389.html. Accessed 23 June 2023.
49. Cook JE, Purdie-Vaughns V, Meyer IH, Busch JTA. Intervening within and across levels: a multilevel approach to stigma and public health. Soc Sci Med. 2014;103:101–9.
50. Hatzenbuehler ML, Phelan JC, Link BG. Stigma as a fundamental cause of population health inequalities. Am J Public Health. 2013;103(5):813–21.
51. Benintendi A, Kosakowski S, Lagisetty P, Larochelle M, Bohnert ASB, Bazzi AR. "I felt like I had a scarlet letter": recurring experiences of structural stigma surrounding opioid tapers among patients with chronic, non-cancer pain. Drug Alcohol Depend. 2021;222:108664.
52. U.S. Department of Health and Human Services. Pain management best practices inter-agency task force report: updates, gaps, inconsistencies, and recommendations. 2019, May. Retrieved June 23, 2023. U. S. Department of Health and Human Services website: https://www.hhs.gov/ash/advisory-committees/pain/reports/index.html
53. Dumit J. Illnesses you have to fight to get: facts as forces in uncertain, emergent illnesses. Soc Sci Med. 2006;62(3):577–90.
54. van Boekel LC, Brouwers EP, van Weeghel J, Garretsen HF. Stigma among health professionals towards patients with substance use disorders and its consequences for healthcare delivery: systematic review. Drug Alcohol Depend. 2013;131(1–2):23–35.
55. Tsai AC, Kiang MV, Barnett ML, Beletsky L, Keyes KM, McGinty EE, Smith LR, Strathdee SA, Wakeman SE, Venkataramani AS. Stigma as a fundamental hindrance to the United States opioid overdose crisis response. PLoS Med. 2019;16(11):e1002969.
56. Waugh OC, Byrne DG, Nicholas MK. Internalized stigma in people living with chronic pain. J Pain. 2014;15(5):550.e1–10.
57. Slade SC, Molloy E, Keating JL. Stigma experienced by people with nonspecific chronic low back pain: a qualitative study. Pain Med. 2009;10(1):143–54.
58. Lagisetty P, Garpestad C, Larkin A, Macleod C, Antoku D, Slat S, Thomas J, Powell V, Bohnert ASB, Lin LA. Identifying individuals with opioid use disorder: validity of international classification of diseases diagnostic codes for opioid use, dependence and abuse. Drug Alcohol Depend. 2021;221:108583.
59. Gavin K. Pain patients who take opioids can't get in the door at half of primary care clinics. Michigan Medicine. 2021, January 25. https://www.michiganmedicine.org/health-lab/pain-patients-who-take-opioids-cant-get-door-half-primary-care-clinics. Accessed 23 June 2023.
60. Lagisetty P, Macleod C, Thomas J, Slat S, Kehne A, Heisler M, Bohnert ASB, Bohnert KM. Assessing reasons for decreased primary care access for individuals on prescribed opioids: an audit study. Pain. 2021;162(5):1379–86.
61. Lagisetty PA, Healy N, Garpestad C, Jannausch M, Tipirneni R, Bohnert ASB. Access to primary care clinics for patients with chronic pain receiving opioids. JAMA Netw Open. 2019;2(7):e196928.
62. Goffman E. Stigma—notes on the management of spoiled identity. Touchstone. 1963. ISBN13: 9780671622442.

63. Fact Sheet Stigma. Pain Mnagement Best Practices Inter-agency Task Force. 2019. Available at: https://www.hhs.gov/sites/defaault/files/pmft-fact-sheet-stigma_508-2019-08-13.pdf Accessed: 07 October 2024.

64. Dowell D, Haegerich TM, Chou R. CDC guideline for prescribing opioids for chronic pain – United States, 2016. MMWR Recomm Rep. 2016;65(1):1–49.

65. Davis CS, Lieberman AJ. Laws limiting prescribing and dispensing opioids in the United States, 1989-2-19. Addiction. 2021;116(7):1817–27

66. Agnoli A, Xing G, Tancredi DJ, Magnan E, Jerant A, Fenton JJ. Association of dose tapering with overdose or mental health crisis among patients prescribed long-term opioids. JAMA. 2021;326(5):411–9. Erratum in: JAMA. 2022 Feb 15;327(7):688. Erratum in: JAMA. 2022 Feb 15;327(7):687.

67. Oliva EM, Bowe T, Manhapra A, Kertesz S, Hah JM, Henderson P, Robinson A, Paik M, Sandbrink F, Gordon AJ, Trafton JA. Associations between stopping prescriptions for opioids, length of opioid treatment, and overdose or suicide deaths in US veterans: observational evaluation. BMJ. 2020;368:m283.

68. Szalavitz M. What the opioid crisis took from people in pain. The New York Times. 2022, March 7.

69. Himmelstein G, Bates D, Zhou L. Examination of stigmatizing language in the electronic health record. JAMA Netw Open. 2022;5(1):e2144967.

70. Kelly JF, Westerhoff CM. Does it matter how we refer to individuals with substance-related conditions? A randomized study of two commonly used terms. Int J Drug Policy. 2010;21(3):202–7.

71. Shipton EE, Bate F, Garrick R, Steketee C, Shipton EA, Visser EJ. Systematic review of pain medicine content, teaching, and assessment in medical school curricula internationally. Pain Ther. 2018;7(2):139–61.

72. Social determinants of health. (2019). WHO - World Health Organization. https://www.who.int/health-topics/social-determinants-of-health#tab=tab_1

73. Dickinson KL, Roberts JD, Banacos N, Neuberger L, Koebele E, Blanch-Hartigan D, Shanahan EA. Structural racism and the COVID-19 experience in the United States. Health Secur. 2021;19(S1):S14–26.

74. Puntillo F, Giglio M, Brienza N, Viswanath O, Urits I, Kaye AD, Pergolizzi J, Paladini A, Varrassi G. Impact of COVID-19 pandemic on chronic pain management: looking for the best way to deliver care. Best Pract Res Clin Anaesthesiol. 2020;34(3):529–37.

75. Artiga S, Hinton E. Beyond health care: the role of social determinants in promoting health and health equity. Kaiser Family Foundation Brief. 2018, May 10.

76. Magnan S. Social determinants of health 101 for health care: five plus five. NAM perspectives. Discussion paper, National Academy of Medicine, Washington, DC; 2017.

77. Marmot MG, Smith GD, Stansfeld S, Patel C, North F, Head J, White I, Brunner E, Feeney A. Health inequalities among British civil servants: the Whitehall II study. Lancet. 1991;337(8754):1387–93.

78. Joynt M, Train MK, Robbins BW, Halterman JS, Caiola E, Fortuna RJ. The impact of neighborhood socioeconomic status and race on the prescribing of opioids in emergency departments throughout the United States. J Gen Intern Med. 2013;28(12):1604–10.

79. Karran EL, Grant AR, Moseley GL. Low back pain and the social determinants of health: a systematic review and narrative synthesis. Pain. 2020;161(11):2476–93.

80. Katz JN. Persistent racial disparities in joint replacement use: commentary on an article by Caroline P. Thirukumaran, MBBS, MHA, PhD, et al.: "geographic variation and disparities in total joint replacement use for medicare beneficiaries: 2009 to 2017". J Bone Joint Surg Am. 2020;102(24):e137.

81. Yap ZL, Summers SJ, Grant AR, Moseley GL, Karran EL. The role of the social determinants of health in outcomes of surgery for low back pain: a systematic review and narrative synthesis. Spine J. 2022;22(5):793–809.

82. Thirukumaran CP, Cai X, Glance LG, Kim Y, Ricciardi BF, Fiscella KA, Li Y. Geographic variation and disparities in total joint replacement use for medicare beneficiaries: 2009 to 2017. J Bone Joint Surg Am. 2020;102(24):2120–8.

83. Fiscella K, Sanders MR. Racial and ethnic disparities in the quality of health care. Annu Rev Public Health. 2016;37:375–94.

84. Delanois RE, Tarazi JM, Wilkie WA, Remily E, Salem HS, Mohamed NS, Pollack AN, Mont MA. Social determinants of health in total knee arthroplasty: are social factors associated with increased 30-day post-discharge cost of care and length of stay? Bone Joint J. 2021;103-B(6 Supple A):113–8.

85. Summers KM, Deska JB, Almaraz SM, Hugenberg K, Lloyd EP. Poverty and pain: low-SES people are believed to be insensitive to pain? J Exp Psychol. 2021;95:104116.

86. Lacey RJ, Campbell P, Lewis M, Protheroe J. The impact of inadequate health literacy in a population with musculoskeletal pain. Health Lit Res Pract. 2018;2(4):e215–20.

87. Rogers AH, Bakhshaie J, Orr MF, Ditre JW, Zvolensky MJ. Health literacy, opioid misuse, and pain experience among adults with chronic pain. Pain Med. 2020;21(4):670–6.

88. Maly A, Vallerand AH. Neighborhood, socioeconomic, and racial influence on chronic pain. Pain Manag Nurs. 2018;19(1):14–22.

89. Mathur VA, Trost Z, Ezenwa MO, Sturgeon JA, Hood AM. Mechanisms of injustice: What we (do not) know about racialized disparities in pain. Pain. 2021;163(6):999–1005.

Ethical Decision Making in Pain Management

9

Ethics and Pain Care

One of the key responsibilities that healthcare professionals have to their patients with pain is the delivery of pain care that is ethical [1] and which pays particular attention to ensuring the care delivered is consistent with the individual patient's wishes and values. Virtually every healthcare professional organization around the world has a mission statement that includes mention of the relationship between ethics and pain management that is similar in spirit to the American Nurses Association's (ANA) position statement titled *The Ethical Responsibility to Manage Pain and the Suffering it Causes* [2], which was written by the ANA Center for Ethics and Human Rights and adopted by the ANA Board of Directors in 2018. At its core, the purpose of this position statement was "*to provide ethical guidance and to support nurses as they fulfill their responsibility to provide optimal care to persons experiencing pain.*" This position statement underscores that nurses have ethical responsibilities which include providing care that attempts to effectively alleviate pain and suffering, using modalities supported by scientific evidence, and take into consideration the use of opioid analgesics in the context of the overdose epidemic our country. Additionally, the position statement emphasizes a patient's right to self-determine, to receive pain care that is respectful, and to receive pain care that is equitable in its availability and delivery regardless of a patient's cultural background, values, or beliefs.

Often the ethical delivery of medical care and practice consists of taking an algorithmic approach to caring for patients. This methodology often facilitates efficiency, continuity, and consistency of care. This model of care might make it seem reasonable for one to presume that regardless of pathophysiologic cause, patients with any specific type of pain are essentially similar to each other, which then allows for a certain degree of reproducibility in pain management approaches as well. In a real-world setting, it is not uncommon for someone presenting with chronic pain-related complaint to often have one or more other chief complaints, each of which warrant an appropriate assessment that includes a focused history, physical

© The Author(s), under exclusive license to Springer Nature Switzerland AG 2024   111
K. L. Zacharoff, P. Migdal, *Pain, Drugs, and Ethics*,
https://doi.org/10.1007/978-3-031-63018-7_9

examination, and laboratory testing which will allow for the ability to make a diagnosis, or at a minimum a differential diagnosis. Once a reasonable degree of diagnostic certainty is achieved, this would then normally be followed by communication to the patient, dialogue with the patient, and formulation of a treatment plan, that is realistic and incorporates both patient and clinician goals and expectations. Next would normally be the process of informed consent, considering and verifying patient understanding of potential risks and benefits of the treatment plan, followed by a trial implementation of that plan. Not dissimilar to medical conditions, there would then be a need to perform routine reassessment(s) of the patient at some point, particularly focused on the failure or success of achieving mutually agreed upon therapeutic goals, and with follow-up visits as necessary to allow for adjustments to the treatment plan as needed over the continuum of care. This approach is relatively simple, in principle easy to apply, often with little disruption to the thought processes of accepted clinical paradigms and heuristics.

When it comes to the assessment and treatment of acute, subacute, and chronic pain, the delivery of ethical pain care may not often be as clear-cut as what is described above, and may frequently be different when compared to other medical conditions in clinically ethical practice for a variety of reasons.

In many cases, the symptom profile associated with subacute or chronic pain may be more subjective than usual and dissociated from objective clinical signs which might typically assist in the identification of the cause(s) of pain, sometimes with patient complaints of pain-related symptoms even after a known injury has occurred and "normal" healing has taken place. In fact, in certain situations, such as chronic pain, objective findings might be difficult or even impossible to identify and affirm a pathophysiologic cause. Patients with chronic pain may have significantly compromised levels of functional capacity, which may also make it difficult to conclude whether the functional impact has led to deconditioning, and whether the deconditioning has actually led to a further decreased tolerance to pain.

Regardless of the unique aspects of pain compared with those of other common medical conditions, when patients seek medical attention for the assessment and treatment of a pain-related condition, from an ethical perspective, they generally present with individual **ethical needs** [3]. These needs often include **being treated with respect, and communication that fosters a sense of dignity and promotes a feeling of integrity** (i.e., being believed). From an ethical perspective, patients may often want to feel that they have an equal role in clinical decision making (some degree of autonomy), that they will not be harmed, but be protected, and that **they will be treated fairly and equally** (regardless of culture, race, gender, etc.). Alternatively, it is also possible that a subset of patients may seek medical attention for pain and to be "told what to do" to manage their pain, in a paternalistic fashion.

There are particular **clinician characteristics** which can help to satisfy the abovementioned ethical needs of patients. Primarily, it is the characteristic of having the capacity to think first about **how pain care can be delivered to the patient in the most ethical and virtuous ways possible.** This generally includes **fostering a sense of relationship with the patient which is trusting** and **communicating with them in a way that conveys a sense of responsibility with accountability**.

Another integral clinician characteristic is the ability to capture that patient's narrative in a manner which assures the patient that the impact of pain on their function and overall quality of life is of paramount importance, and that any measures taken will be the product of a therapeutic alliance as opposed to a paternalistic one.

Several challenges may present with respect to the delivery of ethical pain care [3]. Sometimes these challenges may result in patients suffering from uncontrolled, poorly controlled, and, in many cases, unnecessary pain. Several factors are involved and can fuel the development of this phenomenon. First is that there may often **a failure by many nonexpert frontline practitioners to consider the treatment of pain as a clinical priority**. As mentioned other times throughout this book, few would argue that that while education about the assessment and treatment of other common medical conditions such as diabetes and hypertension is the standard for clinicians in training, education and pain assessment and treatment is often lacking, fragmented, inconsistent, and even absent in many clinical training programs [4, 5]. In many cases, these clinicians may also have never received any formal training about addiction and substance use disorders as well. It is virtually a given that the overwhelming majority of pain treatment plans will likely include a prescription for one or more pharmacologic agents. When clinicians are presented with clinical encounters and conditions for which they have received little or no education, which may also require a deviation from normal (and often "comfortable") practice paradigms, the end result could be **a lack of comfort with respect to prescribing certain analgesic medications, a desire to avoid those clinical situations entirely**, a diminished degree of confidence in managing pain, and ultimately a deficiency of a very important ingredient of an ethical therapeutic relationship—**trust**. This can contribute to the fact that it is not uncommon for patients with a chronic pain-related complaint to feel a lack of trust, a fear of being stigmatized, to be fearful about being believed, and in some cases even ashamed of their pain-related diminished level of functional incapacity [6]. These circumstances can also promote clinicians to exhibit some degree of unethical behavior toward patients in a variety of ways, including discrimination in the form of bias, prejudice, or stigma. Ultimately, the **product may be a poorly functioning clinician-patient relationship.**

Most would agree that the treatment of pain, which includes easing someone's pain-related suffering, ultimately leading to an improvement in function and overall quality of life, is a fundamental ethical right and it is also likely indisputable that clinicians who treat patients with pain have both an ethical duty and moral obligation to do so in a manner that is as effective and safe as possible. Unfortunately, many issues may often present challenges to the ethical treatment of people with pain [3]. In many instances, ethical questions continue today to persist with respect to the importance of pain treatment in frontline clinical practice as compared to other common medical conditions (e.g., hypertension, diabetes, etc.). With pain being one of the most single common reasons that people seek medical attention, one would imagine this would not likely be an issue today given the prevalence of pain in the United States at present, but it in fact it is. There are also lingering questions about where the duties of healthcare professionals begin and end with respect to pain treatment, along with balancing other duties associated with an "imperative" to provide "adequate" pain treatment. There are even questions about defining just what "adequate" means with respect to managing pain and frequently little to no guidance for clinicians about its exact meaning. In some cases, clinicians, health-care systems, and even regulators may consider "adequate" to be an arbitrary percentage of decrease in subjective pain ratings (e.g., numerical rating scale 0–10) such as 30% from initial ratings, without much regard given to the impact of pain on functional capacity and overall quality of life.

The main challenges frequently obstructing the ethical delivery of pain care are numerous, and what follows is in no way a comprehensive list, but more of a representation of the most common barriers [3]. First is that **clinicians, healthcare systems, payers, and other stakeholders may often fail to prioritize the importance of pain treatment in patient care**. This could be in part due to the prevalence of the typical curative, biomedical, mechanistic models that are common in medicine today as opposed to ones that are more patient-centered, focused on more blended physiologic, biopsychosocial, humanistic models. Second is **the frequent inability for clinicians to develop trusting relationships with their patients** because of time constraints and practice models which do not often prioritize continuity of care as a key mission. This may result in a poor level of clinician-patient communication, an increased likelihood of misunderstanding by the patient, the clinician, or both, and a diminished sense by the patient of being believed, all of which are considered to be critical with respect to safely and effectively treating a frequently subjective medical condition like pain. A third barrier, and mentioned many times in this book, is **the frequent lack of foundational knowledge resulting from a lack of clinician education about pain and its management**. Additionally, **fears associated with the "environment" surrounding the use of opioid analgesics and educational deficits about "opioid risk"** including addiction, dependence, tolerance, substance use, and adverse effects. **It is not uncommon for the patient and/or caregiver to express the desire to avoid opioids due to what they have been exposed to in the mainstream media or other sources.** Lastly, is a frequent **lack of consensus with respect to clinician accountability regarding successful pain treatment by healthcare institutions and systems**. In fact, it may be much more likely that there is a greater level of consensus in healthcare systems with respect to the overdose epidemic and its relationship to opioid prescribing and potential cost-saving measures, than to successful pain treatment outcomes.

Prioritization of Pain Care

How pain factors into the prioritization process and a sense of responsibility to the delivery of ethical healthcare may differ based on the particular stakeholder. For example, it is not uncommon for clinicians to report that the complexity and subjective nature of pain and associated patient needs do not often "fit" within a reasonable allocation of time necessary to maintain efficiency within a busy clinical practice. This is especially the case in nonexpert clinical settings, such as Family Medicine and Internal Medicine, etc., who will frequently report that addressing conditions such as hypertension, coronary artery disease, and diabetes demand a higher level of attention. Additionally, clinicians may lack confidence when called upon to assess and treat patients with pain due to educational deficits, and perceived differences in paradigms necessary to effectively do so. At the system level, inter-professional teams and educational initiatives may be inadequate, sometimes being deflected to limit responsibility and/or resource allocation, which in today's health-care systems are often limited. With respect to regulatory agencies, payers, and other similar stakeholders, personal and professional responsibilities are often stressed, which may create an environment of fear of reprisal instead of one that fosters competent, compassionate, and readily available pain care.

In today's healthcare environment, what seems to be lacking is that making pain a priority in caring for patients does *not* seem to be the baseline for a majority of frontline practitioners, healthcare systems, payers, and regulatory agencies. Much of this may be related to the aforementioned "opioid pendulum" which has shifted in the direction of reduced opioid prescribing in an effort to reduce associated over-doses and fatalities regardless of the impact of access to patients in need. Between 2000 and 2010, it was common to find messaging associated with safe and effective prescribing of opioids while "maintaining access" for those considered to be appro-priate candidates for opioid therapy. The importance of maintaining access to opi-oids for appropriate candidates has essentially been removed from messaging at virtually almost every stakeholder level, being replaced by messaging which pro-motes less prescribing, except for a small subset of patients with a diagnosed, objec-tive cause of pain such as cancer-related pain, sickle cell disease-related pain, etc. But that does not mean that there has not been a significant impact of this new mes-saging. It is now often reported that this shift has in many cases made it more diffi-cult for even people with these objective diagnoses to find clinicians willing to prescribe opioids to them [7]. A recent report from the American Medical Association [8] identified that reductions in opioid prescribing have *not* led to reductions in drug-related mortality, and that *"efforts should be made to remove inequities and other barriers for patients with substance use disorders, mental illness, and pain."*

Clinician Relationships with Patients, Communication, and Trust

A patient's life context and their narrative are critical components to the delivery of safe and effective pain care, yet the current economic medical environment in many cases does not support the time and effort it requires to obtain this important information. Most healthcare providers today are quick to report that the amount of time they have to spend with a patient during a clinical visit is typically limited, and that it may seem overly idealistic to think that there is often time available to truly capture a detailed patient's pain-related narrative and context in many cases in a busy clinic setting. Despite its value proposition in healthcare, technology can also present a barrier to the development of a meaningful clinician-patient relationship, effective   communication,   development   of   trust,   and   identification   of patient-centered goals and expectations of pain treatment. Electronic Medical Records (EMRs) and their associated devices and systems can negatively impact the delivery of ethical pain care. With templated assessment forms and time-consuming data entry, the ability to have the medical record reflect an individualized patient narrative can be challenging, unless there is the capability to enter free-text, which can be quite time consuming to enter. Additionally, if a given template does not incorporate certain fields that facilitate capturing this information as identifiable data, it may often remain unqueried, unidentified, and essentially undocumented.

Sir William Osler (1849–1919) wrote in the *Boston Medical and Surgical Journal* [9] that "*it is more important to know what sort of patient has a disease (risk factor or adverse effect) than to know what sort of disease a patient has*." It is important to remember that something as subjective as pain can sometimes lead to lack of belief and even mistrust in certain cases. **Capturing the patient narrative and pain context in terms of their life can be a key ingredient to fostering trust and enhancing communication**. It follows then that this can also contribute to the development of ethical, and mutually-derived, goals of pain treatment, which not surprisingly will likely significantly improve the chance of satisfaction of outcomes.

Lack of Foundational Knowledge and Educational Deficits Regarding Pain

As mentioned previously, basic undergraduate and graduate healthcare professional education programs may often not provide sufficient training for future clinicians that enables them to achieve the delivery of competent, ethical, and compassionate pain care. A lack of knowledge may lead to a poor level of understanding about the complexity of pain, and its intimate relationship with the person experiencing it and the impact that pain can have on that person's life. Additionally, a lack of foundational knowledge may subject clinicians and patients to directives which are based on other factors, which may not necessarily have ethical care as their mission, such as economics, efficiency, and cost-saving measures. This may then create conflict which can potentially degrade levels of satisfaction for all parties involved, including clinician gratification resulting from optimal care delivery and successful pain treatment outcomes. It is important to consider that patient level of knowledge may frequently be deficient as well, despite a plethora of "one-size fits all" information about pain treatment the Internet has to offer. Educational deficits about pain management may set the stage for the use of more mechanistic approaches to pain assessment and treatment which often include unimodal, pharmacologic treatments which may or may not necessarily lead to successful outcomes. Certainly, the use of opioid analgesics as a component of a pain treatment plan has fallen victim to many of these external forces which in in turn may lead to patients being denied access to them for reasons other than ethical ones. Coupled with a lack of education about addiction and substance use disorder, the result may be a desire for clinicians to choose to avoid caring for patients with pain altogether, leaving patients in many cases with no place to turn for pain treatment they need. Patients may perceive these actions as a lack of desire to provide ethical care, leading to decreased levels of empathy, respect, belief, and trust which then may lead to increased suffering and decreased satisfaction.

It is not uncommon for clinicians to carry into their clinical practices approaches that they are most comfortable or familiar with—often those learned during their training. In a way, clinicians might become biased toward these familiar approaches, which sometimes do not necessarily prioritize the best interests of the patient. For certain patients, the reward for seeking medical attention often comes in the form of the prescription of a medication to which they do not have access to "over the counter." There is a high likelihood that before someone seeks medical attention for a pain-related condition, that type(s) of self-treatment has been employed. It is also very often the case that patients with pain might be expecting a paternalistic approach to their treatment, such as the prescription of medication(s) which in many cases in the past would often be opioid analgesics. The intersection of clinician confidence and the utilization of learned modalities and patient expectations for prescribed treatment may potentially corrupt the ethical delivery of pain care. Regardless, from the perspective of both clinicians and patients, all but the most expert-level clinicians may focus entirely on the biomedical treatment of pain without regard to the importance of incorporating biopsychosocial-focused approaches which are more likely to consider the context of an individual's pain and the narrative of how it may be affecting their lives.

Fear, Regulatory Scrutiny, and Pain Management

The phrase "malpractice medicine" often refers to clinical decision-making practices which are based on placing concern about malpractice liability over all other factors which typically inform clinical decisions. This basically means that ethical standards may not be driving healthcare decisions based on safety, efficacy, and autonomous decisions. There are many instances where this defensive type of practice has been identified, such as the overuse of diagnostic radiologic testing with the intention of making sure that there is adequate documentation in the medical record to prevent allegations of negligence, even when from a clinical perspective there is a lack of supporting clinical rationale for testing beyond solely "liability protection." For many clinicians involved in treating patients with pain, a similar phenomenon exists. This arises when there is **a fear of liability and regulatory scrutiny** linked to issues related to the development of tolerance, dependence, addiction, and the risk of overdose. In certain situations, this may result in an override of the standard ethical calculus about how pain should be managed in the best interests of the patient, especially when opioid analgesics could potentially be an appropriate component of a pain treatment plan. A significant level of negative publicity and attention has been paid to the use of opioid analgesics in federal, state, and local authority messaging with respect to the prescribing of opioids, and the overdose epidemic plaguing the United States has in certain cases negatively impacted the clinican's ability to delivery ethical pain care.

Additionally, in the case of prescribing controlled substances such as opioid analgesics for pain, the ethical calculus is different from other clinical situations. **Informed consent** typically refers to a process which includes demonstration that there is a risk/benefit analysis performed, which is then discussed with the patient. There is also a requirement that there be demonstration that this analysis and information is understood by the patient, ultimately allowing them to make the most informed decision possible. This incorporates the idea that the clinician and patient have communicated about **patient-level risks and benefits**. From a regulatory perspective at the time of this writing, a pain treatment risk/benefit analysis and informed consent process must now also include consideration of and communication about **risks to people other than the patient**. For example, if an opioid is prescribed, there needs to be consideration of risks related to **other members of the household** who might come into contact with or be exposed to the opioid, **other people who have access to the home or dwelling where the patient resides**, such as members of the community, and **risks to society at large.** This means that in addition to determining, communicating, and demonstrating understanding about specific risks to the patient, the informed consent process and the safety and efficacy profile considers potential harm to others. Inattention to these details may lead to punitive regulatory consequences for prescribing clinicians.

From a regulatory perspective, another complicating factor contributing to promoting a fear of regulatory scrutiny among clinicians may arise from state-run Prescription Drug Monitoring Program data, which refers to data stored in a database which tracks prescriptions written for controlled substances such as opioid analgesics. Most people consider the main purpose of these databases to be as a tool intended to combat the overdose epidemic, helping to identify people who may be seeking and filling prescriptions for medications like opioid analgesics from multiple healthcare professionals, often referred to as "drug-seeking" or "doctor shopping." But in addition to capturing this data, these databases also have the capability to keep track of prescriptions written by individual prescribers and can identify prescribing patterns which can then be measured against those from similar-specialty clinicians in the same geographic region. The intention here is to detect prescribers who fall "outside the normal range" for their specific discipline or who deviate significantly from the individual state departments of health guidelines or recommendations, a form of profiling. This means that someone who is caring for a patient who may require a higher dosage or more doses than usual might trigger a "red flag" and ultimately result in the generation of a warning to the clinician from the state medical board, the DEA, or both. These can cause clinicians to feel fearful about being labeled as a "high prescriber," which may then result in reluctance to prescribe the opioids in those doses or quantities to patients who need them, which in turn has the potential to corrupt the ethical delivery of pain care.

Unfortunately, fear of regulatory scrutiny has created an atmosphere in the clinical environment that in some cases seems *anything but* ethical. It is now not uncommon to hear about clinicians seeking to avoid putting themselves in these types of situations by proactively letting patients with pain know that opioids would not be prescribed in certain medical practices or clinical settings, often leaving patients in need feeling that they have nowhere to turn. In other cases, there may be a fear that people in need of opioid therapy but denied access might choose to obtain them from illicit channels of distribution, which could potentially be tragic, especially if they are counterfeit medication preparations which could be contaminated with synthetic substances like fentanyl.

Another example of the potential negative consequences of the dynamic that exists today is illustrated in an editorial that appeared in the *New York Times* in March 2022 titled *What the Opioid Crisis Took from People in Pain* [10], which detailed the case of a patient with chronic pain related to objective medical causes (multiple trauma) being told despite his protest that his longstanding opioid doses were going to suddenly be decreased by half, presumably to avoid being the clinician being "flagged" for inappropriate prescribing. When denied the usual dose of opioids which had been prescribed for years, the patient committed suicide, and his family successfully sued the clinician for malpractice.

Ethical Perspective

Patients have an ethical and moral right to treatment for pain and unnecessary associated suffering. Clinicians have an ethical and moral duty to provide or at a minimum facilitate such treatment. It is incumbent upon clinicians to be responsible to do three things with respect to the ethical practice of pain care. First, and most obviously, is an obligation to **avoid inflicting further pain and suffering** beyond that which is necessary in order to provide evidence-based pain care. Second is a responsibility to do all that can be done within the current limits of knowledge, scientific evidence, and available resources **to help patients to relieve their pain and associated suffering**. This responsibility is not limited to merely decreasing someone's pain rating, but more importantly to **help maintain or improve their level of function and overall quality of life** in the face of the pain they are experiencing. Thirdly, it is of the utmost importance that **the context of the patient's pain, their narrative, and their individuality be considered** when helping them to find a path forward, meaning that there are no likely "cookie-cutter" approaches to managing one person's pain.

There are multiple drivers of clinical ethical decision-making, which may be cognitive or precognitive, and conscious or unconscious. While they are most often rooted in a desire to "do no harm," it is reasonable to consider that clinical decisions are often based on limitations of knowledge, where clinicians typically recommend what they are familiar with, or what they know, and sometimes based on prior experiences. The core ethical principles, **autonomy, justice, nonmaleficence, and beneficence** should drive clinical decisions as well. Implementing ethical decisions may or may not be simple.

It is important to remember that when treating someone's pain, **the person with pain has the right to be a contributor in the determination of defining and identifying what a "successful treatment outcome" is**. In fact, some have proposed that patient satisfaction may be the only "true" desired pain treatment outcome [11], acknowledging that it can be a complicated concept which is intimately related to often predetermined goals and expectations. Some consider patient satisfaction to be the *only* important pain treatment outcome, while others consider the patient's narrative and successfully treating the factors of the patient's life that pain affects to be of utmost importance [12]. Since 2000, there has been much deliberation to consider the pathophysiologic or "**mechanistic approach**," to be the most crucial factor to consider for pain treatment, which relies on the ethical duty to only provide treatments that are appropriate and known to be effective for a given pain mechanism. Alternatively, many have argued that a more "**humanistic approach**" takes into consideration not only the physical, but also the biopsychosocial aspects of pain as well. What is most important in helping to define pain treatment planning and success lies in the pain assessment process. This involves **mutual clinician and patient determination of goals and expectations of pain treatment** which are individualized *not only* to the patient, but also to the clinician. This takes into consideration the patient's context, the patient's needs, and also the clinician's knowledge, comfort levels, and perspectives. This is also an opportunity not only for patients to describe their particular needs and desires, but also for clinicians to disclose to patients the constraints which they may be subjected to (e.g., from an institutional or regulatory policy or guideline) which could potentially negatively impact ethical delivery of pain care if left undisclosed. This information is important for clinicians to communicate to patients in an effort to neutralize the perception of what might be considered to be potentially punitive measures, such as the use of risk mitigation strategies such as urine drug screening, accessing the PDMP, and opioid agreements. All of this can potentially contribute to the ability to provide ethical pain care to the greatest extent possible.

Additionally, it is important to consider that unlike the "opioid pendulum" which has moved from what many refer to as a period of overly liberal prescribing of opioids to one where opioid prescribing is discouraged, **there is no "ethical pendulum."** This translates to the idea that regardless of the myriad of forces at play in terms of the role that opioid analgesic prescribing has in the management of pain, **ethical pain care still must be delivered,** with compassion, empathy, and understanding. In the early 2000s, regulatory messaging reinforced the idea that careful opioid prescribing included a duty to ensure maintaining access to these medications who were considered to be appropriate candidates for them as a part of a pain treatment plan. With the rise of opioid-related overdose deaths, the message of maintaining access seems to have diminished and, in many cases, disappeared, often now leaving clinicians with conflicting thoughts about their role in perpetuating the overdose epidemic and how to deliver pain care as ethically as possible.

By definition, **ethical pain care** means that there is consideration of the delicate balance of efficacy and safety of any treatment options that are considered as potential components of a pain treatment plan. As will be detailed in the chapters following, ethical care means that patients have the ability to participate in the decision-making process of the most appropriate course(s) of treatment. The patient's participation should be with a significant **degree of autonomy** that is not unlike that in patients with any other medical condition and its treatment(s). The options presented to the patient should include *all* available options **equitably,**

within the limits of the law, with clear and easy to understand presentation and demonstration of understanding of associated risks and benefits to ensure the ability to participate in making the most informed decision possible. These options should demonstrate the ability to **benefit the patient** in a manner that does not create an **unnecessary or inappropriate level of harm to the patient or others.** These principles do not change with time. As demonstrated above, the end result of so many different forces may result in the delivery of pain care which potentially may leave pain often under- or untreated, which is *not* ethical. This has the potential to be further magnified for disparate patient populations, including minorities, those of lower socio-economic status, the elderly, children, cognitively impaired individuals, and those nearing the end of life, to name a few.

It may be that there needs to be a **recalibration of pain care which relies on ethical decision making as its guide**, care not impacted by other variables, such as public policy or newly released practice recommendations and guidelines. This does not imply that safety, risks, and even efficacy are not dynamic in certain ways; they certainly might be. It is of paramount importance to consider risks posed to people other than the patient in situations where opioid analgesics are considered as part of a pain treatment plan. In addition to patient level risk, risks to other members of the household, the community at large, and even overall societal impact should routinely be considered as part of any ethically derived pain treatment risk/benefit analysis. However, this recalibration must also include education about pain and substance use disorders, to foster presenting treatment choices to patients and their caregivers that are founded on mutually determined, realistic goals and expectations which are ethically sound as well.

Pharmacologic agents are commonly utilized or considered as part of a treatment plan for the majority of patients who present with chronic pain. It is important to consider that among the many challenges which exist with respect to the delivery of ethical pain care detailed above have in some cases been the result of reactive changes in access to certain treatments like opioid analgesics. This has occurred even in the absence of evidence for utilizing other pain treatment options. In some cases, alternative nonopioid pharmacologic treatment options have risk/benefit profiles which *may or may not* be safer or more efficacious than opioids. Simply selecting or offering alternatives to opioids that are not based on scientific evidence, with only considering these alternatives because they are nonopioid, *does not* satisfy a mandate to provide ethical care. The mission to relieve pain and associated suffering is much more complicated than that. There are situations where these principles may overlap, and even sometimes conflict with each other, and an obvious mechanism for weighing and balancing ethical conflict may be unclear. But *it is worth the effort.*

References

1. Jukić M, Puljak L. Legal and ethical aspects of pain management. Acta Med Acad. 2018;47(1):18–26.
2. American Nurses Association. The ethical responsibility to manage pain and the suffering it causes. ANA Position Statement. 2018, February 23. https://www.nursingworld.org/practice-policy/nursing-excellence/official-position-statements/id/

the-ethical-responsibility-to-manage-pain-and-the-suffering-it-causes/.   Accessed   26
June 2023.

3. Carvalho AS, Martins Pereira S, Jácomo A, Magalhães S, Araújo J, Hernández-Marrero P, Costa Gomes C, Schatman ME. Ethical decision making in pain management: a conceptual framework. J Pain Res. 2018;11:967–76.

4. Mezei L, Murinson BB. Johns Hopkins pain curriculum development team. Pain education in North American medical schools. J Pain. 2011;12(12):1199–208.

5. Shipton EE, Bate F, Garrick R, Steketee C, Shipton EA, Visser EJ. Systematic review of pain medicine content, teaching, and assessment in medical school curricula internationally. Pain Ther. 2018;7(2):139–61.

6. Buchman DZ, Ho A, Illes J. You present like a drug addict: patient and clinician perspectives on trust and trustworthiness in chronic pain management. Pain Med. 2016;17(8):1394–406.

7. DeShazer W. 'On that edge of fear': one woman's struggle with sickle cell pain. The New York Times. 2021, May 30.

8. The American Medical Association. Physicians' actions to help end the nation's drug-related overdose and death epidemic—and what still needs to be done. 2023. https://end-overdose-epidemic.org/. Accessed 22 June 2024.

9. John M. From Osler to the cone technique. HSR Proc Intensive Care Cardiovasc Anesth. 2013;5(1):57–8.

10. Szalavitz M. What the opioid crisis took from people in pain. The New York Times. 2022, March 7.

11. Ballantyne JC, Fleisher LA. Ethical issues in opioid prescribing for chronic pain. Pain. 2010;148(3):365–7.

12. Cohen MJ, Jangro WC. A clinical ethics approach to opioid treatment of chronic noncancer pain. AMA J Ethics. 2015;17(6):521–9.

Autonomy

10

The process of informed consent in health care refers to the process of educating a patient with decision-making capacity about potential risks, benefits, and alternatives to a given procedure or medical intervention of any kind [1]. Clinicians have an ethical obligation toward obtaining informed consent that is founded on the idea that patients have an implicit right to direct what happens to them, and that they are able to demonstrate a sufficient level of understanding of these risks, benefits, and viable alternative options. This process should be collaborative in nature, and not coercive in any way. Modern medical ethics provides a mechanism for reproducible and systematic approaches to the practice of medicine, especially to those that may be particularly challenging. This is particularly important in the management of patients with pain, because although context and individuality will likely make every person's pain a unique experience, there needs to be some way to organize approaches toward informed consent and the delivery of pain care.

Patient Autonomy

Many clinicians and ethicists consider **patient autonomy** to be the most important and foundational component of the four principles of modern medical ethics. It is widely accepted that any action taken toward a patient without their explicit consent is considered to be an act of assault, battery, or both, ultimately causing harm to the patient. In its simplest definition, **autonomy is defined as the ability of patients to make their own healthcare decisions and to be able to understand and communicate their understanding sufficiently to those providing their care** [2]. The relationship between autonomy and informed consent is intimate and bidirectional, with informed consent being an unconditional requirement of autonomous decision-making and vice versa. A person's pain is a personal experience and potentially impacts multiple aspects of daily life, which often include the ability to work, maintain social activities, and participate in recreational activities; it is possible (and likely) that patients with pain experience a certain degree of suffering as well.

© The Author(s), under exclusive license to Springer Nature Switzerland AG 2024
K. L. Zacharoff, P. Migdal, *Pain, Drugs, and Ethics*,
https://doi.org/10.1007/978-3-031-63018-7_10

Sometimes pain-related suffering can be overwhelming, and the patient may need significant assitance with the shared decision-making process and making autonomous decisions. **The responsibility to provide this assistance often falls on the shoulders of the clinician**, helping the patient digest and understand the scientific evidence, and giving them the ability to make autonomous decisions that coincide with their individual beliefs, values, goals, and expectations of pain treatment recommendations [3]. Patients also have a responsibility to actively participate in making healthcare-related decisions which align with their individual values and beliefs. In fact, a high level of patient responsibility and engagement has the potential to increase the likelihood of adherence to a mutually-determined pain treatment plan.

Needing a caregiver does not negate a person's capacity for making autonomous decisions about their pain care. It is likely that other people may often play a role in the patient's life as caregivers, helping to maintain patient autonomy, such as close family members, friends, neighbors, etc. This can be particularly important when discussing the goals and expectations of pain care, keeping in mind that patients and their caregivers have a key role in determining the success or failure of a pain treatment plan. It is possible that patients may only be considering a reduction in their pain rating as a metric for determining successful outcomes, and they may need an educational recalibration to additionally consider improvements in overall quality of life and functional capacity as realistic goals of pain treatment. When treating patients with chronic pain, it can also be important to set appropriate expectations about the lower likelihood of a "cure," helping them instead to focus on amelioration of pain rating and pain impact as targets. As long as this education is not coercive, it should be considered to be an important and routine ingredient of autonomous and realistic decision-making and informed consent.

Patient autonomy may be impacted by factors other than their chief pain-related complaint, which should be probed for and considered during the pain assessment process. Similar to the uniqueness of the patient's narrative and the personal context of pain in their life, **a patient's value system and beliefs are likely to be well-formed constructs, and should not be discounted during the patient encounters**. In fact, they can be crucial to helping the patient in the process of identifying goals and expectations of treatment as well. The patient narrative and personal context may also be crucial to the treatment planning from a practical perspective. Patients desiring to avoid pharmacologic therapy, for example, may still desire to do so even after the informed consent process has taken place, and should be respected. Alternatively, patients who express the desire to avoid physical treatment approaches despite demonstrating an understanding of their potential value proposition have an autonomous right for those wishes to be respected as well.

Other factors worthy of consideration that can be of paramount importance are **the patient's level of health literacy, numeracy, and potential barriers to effective communication and comprehension, such as language spoken and cultural identity.** Effectively achieving understanding is the foundational goal of informed consent and autonomous decision-making and requires that discussions take place in a fashion which considers the patient's ability to digest information presented to them. **Avoiding jargon and difficult to understand terms and statistics** is important, but it is no less important than striving to find the "right" level of patient communication of information comprehension. It is possible that depending on their level of health literacy, even a patient's definition of what it means to be "healthy" can vary dramatically, in addition to their definitions of suffering and flourishing [3].

It is also important to be aware that social norms with respect to pain and its management may vary from patient to patient based on their cultural and religious backgrounds. Sometimes this may also be influenced by patient-family dynamics, which can interfere with the informed consent process. For example, it may seem appropriate or convenient to have a family member act as an interpreter when language is a barrier to effective communication and understanding. However, this may present unexpected challenges and corruption of the autonomous process due to the possibility of increased emotionality and/or stress due to the clinical circumstances, the embarrassing nature of information discussed, and even sometimes biases the family member may have related to their own opinions about pain management and decision-making. Awareness of these and other variables at the patient level and their potential impact on pain treatment should be considered to be no less of a duty to maintain and facilitate patient autonomy than any other ethical clinical obligation. Clinicians have a legal and ethical responsibility to treat patients with pain equally in *all* cases [4], providing information, ensuring understanding, and allowing for autonomous decision-making for all patients with the capacity to do so.

Autonomy and the Truth

It is possible for a variety of reasons that conflicts may arise related to a pain diagnosis and possible treatment options: situations where a patient with decision-making capacity does not want to be made aware of a diagnosis, and/or to be involved in the treatment planning process, delegating these roles to a surrogate decision-maker. At first glance, this may be interpreted as an infringement of autonomy, based on the basic human "right to know" or not telling a patient with capacity the truth. In fact, it should be remembered that patient autonomy also encompasses the ability of a patient to make decisions such as this based on a number of possible factors, including but not limited to their cultural background, family dynamics, and desire to maintain hope, etc. It is equally important to avoid precognitively presuming that these desires exist based on a patient's cultural identity based on past clinical experiences with patients of similar cultural background. It is important to identify the patient's wishes and assess the situation on a case-by-case basis, without presumption. It is possible that patient preferences may deviate from other patients of similar cultural, social, religious, and familial contexts and backgrounds.

In order to ensure autonomous decision-making and conduct an accurate assessment that considers the appropriateness of telling a patient the truth while maintaining autonomy when they express a desire "not to know," it is critical to listen, acknowledge, empathize, relate, and offer suggestions that maintain an open dialogue but also respect the patient's wishes [4]. This should be sufficiently documented in the medical record and conveyed to other medical professionals who are members of the care team to ensure that the patient's wishes are adhered to. It is also important to consider that autonomous decision-making and expressed wishes with respect to disclosure and truth-telling may sometimes be dynamic, and that these desires should be carefully revisited and reassessed periodically along the continuum of pain care.

Autonomy, Paternalism, and Medical Decision-Making

Paternalistic medical care is traditionally defined as care and resource allocation that is performed with the intent of promoting the well-being of the patient based on the clinician's opinion and position of authority, without a patient's informed consent. There are many instances of clinical situations when medical decisions are typically made by a clinician, unilaterally and without the patient's input or specific consent [5]. Examples of common paternalistic clinical actions include the ordering of routine diagnostic testing (e.g., laboratory testing), or obtaining consultations with expert clinicians, etc. Typically, when it comes to treatment planning, shared decision-making overrides paternalism in all but the most emergent situations, as a paternalistic approach does not facilitate the ability for a patient to feel respected and to make informed, autonomous decisions. It has been shown that patient participation in therapeutic planning is more likely to yield outcomes which include greater satisfaction, a higher level of pain coping, and overall increased quality of life.

Many patients with a pain-related medical condition or chief complaint often present to their clinical encounter with a relatively simple and passive request—"I don't care, just tell me what I have to do, and just 'get rid' of my pain." It is also not unusual for patients to be told by their clinicians what to do to alleviate their pain without the abovementioned ethically appropriate considerations regarding paternalism, informed consent, etc., and to relate to the patient to "just do what I say." Both these situations may result in varying degrees of "short-circuiting" a shared decision-making process, which is the very hallmark of autonomy and self-determination of medical care. In some cases, it is possible that patients who are suffering significantly from their pain, might not be able to appropriately focus, digest information, demonstrate understanding, and, in some situations, be able to participate in the decision making process at all. In other cases, it is reasonable to expect that a patient has employed some measures of pain control *prior* to seeking medical attention which have been unsuccessful, and the patient is seeking medical attention because they feel that they need access to something "stronger" that can only be obtained by prescription. To a certain degree, patients may present expecting there to be some degree of paternalism in the pain treatment planning process in those circumstances—something less than balanced in terms of shared decision-making. Alternatively, clinicians may sometimes rely on empiric clinical expertise and past experiences to "guide" patients toward certain options, and away from others. This has been described as "relative paternalism," which refers to situations where completely shared decision-making does not necessarily serve the pain patient's best interests. Things can become more complex with respect to the utilization of opioid therapy in pain treatment planning, due to the substantial number of external forces which may potentially influence the offering of opioids as a possible choice for pain control. Clinicians may default to avoiding prescribing opioids due to practice policies which may not necessarily consider the patient's best interests in individual clinical situations, and patients may default to not wanting to be prescribed an opioid because of "fear of addiction" as well.

Patient-centered care is considered to be the norm in modern medical practice and applies to the assessment and management of pain as well. The presumption is that there is active participation from both the clinician and the patient, which ultimately yields mutual agreement in the path forward [6] and considers realistic goals and expectations of both patient and clinician. This does not mean that there may not be some degree of negotiation to achieve agreement. In some cases, the expertise of the clinician may factor into the decision process unequally, and in others the preferences and desires of the patient may carry more weight. However, it is important to consider that how the clinician frames the presentation of information to the patient with pain may potentially influence the patient's level of participation and/or decision-making. In some cases, a clinician's desire to avoid a paternalistic approach to care may sometimes conflict or compete with the best interests of the patient.

One approach to navigating potential paternalistic conflicts is for the clinician to explore the patient's life context to the greatest degree possible, including activities of daily living, potential or existing stressors, and social interactions. This facilitates the potential to allow for the highest level of individualized sharing of information possible to allow the patient to make informed decisions. This is referred to as *patient-preference-satisfaction paternalism* [6], and involves active listening, interpretation, and deliberation, along with careful analysis of the most likely patient preferences based on this analysis. The authority of the clinician remains in place, but not in a coercive fashion. It should also be noted that there may be cases where a patient's preferences do not align with the clinician's impressions or recommendations. This illustrates the point that this type of approach can be a highly dynamic one, as opposed to a purely static paternalistic approach. It is possible and even likely that clinicians may frequently exert some degree of paternalistic behavior during the shared decision-making process. What is of vital importance is that the clinician maintains a respectful, open, and informative manner which considers the likelihood of patient motivation and adherence to a mutually agreed-upon pain treatment plan. It is always possible that the patient may "fail" in one or both these regards. Their expected level of motivation may fall short, their ability to adhere to a treatment plan may fall short as well. This means that the clinician needs to let the patient know that in the event that one or both of these situations arise, that in a collaborative way, alternative approaches to pain treatment will be considered, offered, and discussed without retribution or dismissal.

It is reasonable to conclude that completely mutual decision-making in pain treatment planning is the most desirable approach, although it may not necessarily always be the most practical one. Some may consider autonomous decision-making and paternalistic pain care to be polar opposites of each other, positing that any degree of paternalism implies that the patient is incapable of making a decision that considers their best interests. In fact, it is possible that "protecting" a patient from any degree of paternalistic pain care may inadvertently lead to increased pain, anxiety, and associated suffering [7]. Having an approach that prioritizes patient autonomy, without dictating it strictly in the absence of considering other ethical principles (beneficence, nonmaleficence, justice), is a much more realistic and ethical route to take.

Clinician Autonomy

A survey of clinicians in the United States today would likely reveal that most feel that to some degree their ability to treat patients with pain in a clinically autonomous fashion has been significantly compromised and diminished since 2000. In fact, it is likely that many clinicians of virtually all healthcare disciplines would express that they have in many ways lost the ability to voice their opinions about making pain management decisions that are based primarily on *patient welfare, patient autonomy, and social justice*—the three main components of the American Board of Internal Medicine's "*A Physician's Charter*" [8]. Possible reasons for the high prevalence of these perceptions include an increasing number of pain management-related practice recommendations and/or guidelines, which have been at times incongruous with the clinically ethical mission of pain treatment, not necessarily aligned with delivering compassionate pain care and alleviating suffering, and sometimes inconsistent with each other in their messaging about best practices as well. Certainly, a lack of substantial scientific evidence basis about the role of opioid analgesics in pain management has been a signifiant contributor as well. Since 2000, when pain was designated the 5th vital sign, and the subsequent decade was designated to be the *Decade of Pain Control and Research*, the consensus seemed to be that the mission was to prioritize conducting research necessary to provide scientific evidence to support pain management decision-making, especially if opioids were considered for long-term pain treatment. Unfortunately, this did not happen, partly because the management of pain does not live in a vacuum, and also because of many other developments.

A noteworthy development related to the abovementioned mission of pain care was the ensuing "opioid epidemic." It was not uncommon in the late 1990s for clinicians to be vulnerable to successful litigation for malpractice for undertreating patients with pain. Without a substantial educational foundation, clinicians responded to this vulnerability and desire to treat patients with pain with their prescription pads; often utilizing opioid analgesics as a major component of a pain treatment plan. In fact, clinicians' opioid prescribing increased significantly between 2000 and 2010, which directly correlated with increased incidents of opioid-related overdoses, and overdose fatalities. Retrospectively, there has a lot of finger-pointing with respect to this close correlation. Many have argued that the relationship was a causal one, and that it is abundantly clear that opioids were "overprescribed," without concern for potential aberrant drug-related use, addiction, overdose, etc. Others blame the pharmaceutical companies who manufactured opioids, aggressively marketing them as safe, largely nonaddictive, and compassionate and important available tools to treat pain. Many of these and other controversies continue to exist and to be passionately debated today, with a clear delineation of ideologies of those who feel that opioid analgesics should rarely be prescribed, even for many acute pain patients, and others vehemently arguing that patients with pain are paying an unnecessary price for substance users, and being denied opioid analgesic prescribing due to what is now referred to as the "overdose epidemic" as opposed to the opioid epidemic.

Regardless of the cause(s), it is often not uncommon for the overdose epidemic and concerns about public health and safety to engage regulators, lawmakers, and healthcare systems to step in and implement tactics and strategies designed to modify clinical practice, beliefs, and behaviors when necessary. However, in this case what *was* uncommon is that there was a consensus (sometimes inconsistent) that opioid prescribing needed to change (*in a downward direction*) in order for the opioid/overdose epidemic to be mitigated successfully. Examples of these tactics and strategies are numerous. One of these approaches was the federal mandate that every state needed to develop and implement a Prescription Drug Monitoring Program (PDMP), which would not only monitor what controlled substances were being prescribed to patients to identify medication-seeking behaviors, but also monitor prescribing practices of individual clinicians' prescribing patterns, which could then be flagged for being outside of normal range for a given type of practitioner (e.g., Primary Care) resulting in a report to the state medical board with that information which could then lead to anything from an electronic citation, generation of a prescriber warning letter, an investigation by authorities, etc. Another approach implemented by many state medical boards was a restriction of the quantity, duration, and daily dosage of opioids that could be prescribed by nonexpert clinicians (i.e., *not* pain specialists). In many cases, these restrictions were adopted by state medical boards based on the recommendation in *the 2016 CDC Guideline for Prescribing Opioids for Chronic Pain* [9]. The Drug Enforcement Administration (DEA) also established a commitment to decrease the allowable quantity of opioid medications that could be manufactured and distributed, presumably in an effort to discourage "overprescribing." This is in no way a comprehensive list, but just some illustrations of efforts which were taken to influence clinical practice related to opioid prescribing.

What may not have been taken into consideration by these well-intentioned regulatory "external controls" was their potential impact on how patients with pain who were either dependent on opioid analgesics or potentially appropriate candidates for them might be affected by these changes which were not originating from practicing clinicians making clinical decisions in an autonomously. In fact, many clinicians were of the opinion that these "third parties" were in many ways corrupting the ethically autonomous clinician-patient relationship, with little or no concern for the individual pain-patient's concerns, awareness, or wishes. This is also despite the fact that both clinician *and* patient education was universally considered to be one of the most important strategies for opioid risk mitigation in pain management. In most cases, clinician educational programming was not implemented beyond continuing medical education activities for clinicians in practice, which were often considered to be biased in their messaging because of the fact that in many cases, they were funded in part or supported in total by pharmaceutical companies, notably manufacturers of opioids.

Irrespective of a clinician's autonomy to make informed decisions about which patients might be considered to be appropriate candidates for opioid analgesic trial and therapy, the message sent to clinicians was clear—that *the most effective methodology to stem the tide of the overdose epidemic was considered to be to prescribe fewer opioids.* This led to clinician fear of regulatory scrutiny, in many cases overriding autonomous clinical decision-making which might have in some cases been in the patient's best interests in terms of pain, suffering, and overall quality of life. This also had the potential to negatively impact patient autonomy about their own pain treatment choices as well. In the virtual absence of foundational education, clinicians were and continue today to be forced to make sometimes uninformed decisions about the rationale of prescribing fewer opioids, especially in the absence of recommendations for safe and effective alternatives. In some cases, the effect on access to opioid prescribing has been chilling, with many nonexpert practitioners making the decision to stop prescribing opioid analgesics altogether in their practice, in some cases effectively cutting patients off from access to their opioid medications [10]. In other cases, clinicians responded to the external controls by forcibly tapering prescribed opioid dosages to "fit" within the recommended ceilings put forth by the state and/or clinic restrictions which were often based on the above-mentioned 2016 CDC Guidelines. This is not to say that there were not clinicians who perceived a higher risk of harm to patients after being exposed to these limitations, but there have also been many who wanted to avoid the risk to their licenses and retribution. Many stories began to appear in the mainstream media about clinicians who continued to exceed the recommended limits in their prescribing practices and suffered negative regulatory consequences in varying degrees as a result, including being sent to prison [11].

The relationship between clinician and patient autonomy is intimate and bidirectional. Something to consider is the idea that most often the clinician's role is to help the patient understand the potential risks and benefits of proposed treatments and to help them make autonomous decisions if they have the capacity to do so, after demonstrating understanding of those risks and benefits—once again, referring to the informed consent process. Coincident with the 2016 CDC Guidelines was the fact that in addition to considering *patient-level risk,* clinicians now needed to factor into the equation that when prescribing controlled substances like opioid analgesics, risks beyond those to the patient needed to be considered by the prescriber. These include potential risks to other members of the household who might intentionally or unintentionally be exposed to access to the opioids and suffer consequences as a result, **risks to members of the community** who might gain access to the opioids because of their access to the home, and **risks to members of society** who might gain access as to them as well. Clinicians now needed to inquire about past or present substance use not only of the patient, but also of other people who might have access. Once again, all this taking place without a consistent and wide-ranging educational platform, meaning that clinicians were much more likely to be aware of possible regulatory scrutiny, and less likely to be aware of this "new risk/benefit analysis formula." The end result was that in many cases, it would just be easier for clinicians to avoid the potential hazards of opioid prescribing altogether without necessarily considering the potential impact on patient autonomy. For many patients who were completely adherent to prescribed opioid regimens, this has been bewildering, anguishing, and often frustrating.

Much has been written about possible negative consequences related to unilateral decisions to refuse to refill, refuse to prescribe, or forcibly taper patients who are already on long-term opioid therapy [12]. These negative outcomes vary and range from increased incidence of mental health crises (e.g., anxiety, depression) to suicide, and in some cases, even an increased incidence of drug-related overdose [13]. It is possible that efforts intended to mitigate harm resulting from "liberal" opioid prescribing may have these and other potential unintended negative consequences, most notably denying access to those patients in pain and in need. Again, it is important to point out that most of this was frequently taking place in the absence of clinician education, patient education, or both, resulting in poorly informed decision-making and dramatically decreased levels of both patient and clinician autonomy.

There have been many efforts in recent years to try to reverse these trends and to reduce clinician fears of regulatory scrutiny and practices which could potentially corrupt autonomous pain care. In 2022, the CDC released a revised and updated set of opioid guidelines titled *CDC Clinical Practice Guideline for Prescribing Opioids for Pain—United States, 2022* [14]. This latest version of the CDC guidelines underscored the idea that their intention was to "*improve communication between clinicians and patients about the benefits and risks of pain treatments, including opioid therapy.*" Notably, this new set of guidelines removed specific thresholds for opioid prescribing dosages mentioned in the 2016 CDC guidelines, likely in an effort to try to prevent some of the harms mentioned above resulting from decreased access and forced tapering. In June of 2022, the Supreme Court also clarified its stance on the liability of, and prosecution of, clinicians who were accused of writing "improper prescriptions" for controlled substances which "did not conform to usual professional practice." This decision by the court stated that prosecutors would need to *prove* that a clinician intentionally wrote prescriptions without any legitimate medical purpose.

It remains to be seen as to whether or not the infringement on patient and clinician autonomy with respect to opioid analgesic therapy can (or should) be reversed to some extent, if at all. In its *2021 Overdose Epidemic Report* [15], the American Medical Association (AMA) reported that reductions in opioid prescribing did not in fact lead to reductions of drug-related mortality in the United States. Additionally, in response to opportunity to provide commentary on the public draft of the 2022 CDC Guidelines [16] (Docket No. CDC- 2022-0024), the AMA asked the CDC to "*join the AMA in urging all relevant state, national and federal stakeholders, including legislatures, regulators, health plans, pharmacy chains, and pharmacy benefit management companies (PBMs) to remove all vestiges of inflexible numeric thresholds based on the 2016 Guideline*." In this commentary, the AMA also called for the undertaking of a nation-wide campaign to emphasize that the 2022 CDC guidelines should not be considered as a replacement for autonomous clinical judgment or individualized, self-directed, patient-centered care, urging that the CDC urge the removal of all policies that do not ultimately support "individualized patient care decisions."

There is a delicate balance which needs to be achieved with respect to the mindset that clinicians are able to manage patients with pain with the same level of autonomy that they have afforded to them when treating patients with other medical conditions. Certainly, achieving this goal involves educational efforts which likely best begin for clinicians during their training, so they can incorporate their learning into clinical practices as safely and effectively as possible. Safe practices, much like the use of seatbelts in automobiles, **need to become habits instead of reactions** to fear of scrutiny, low levels of confidence, and public and regulatory opinion. Additionally, this education needs to incorporate learning about the best alternatives to opioid analgesics when appropriate, and needs to be embraced by all stakeholders, especially insurers, healthcare systems, and clinic settings.

If clinicians are not educated about a "plan B" to opioid therapy that is readily available, or are unclear about how to determine what a suitable alternative might be, their ability to offer alternative pain treatment options as part of an autonomous informed consent process could be compromised. Education should include other pharmacologic agents, such as nonopioid pain medications, and other adjunctive medications which could be opioid sparing, such as anticonvulsants, antidepressants, muscle relaxants, etc. Education about other treatment modalities should also be included, which includes interventional treatments, such as neuromodulation and injections, and restorative therapies, such as physical and occupational therapy. Complementary and alternative treatments, such as acupuncture and massage, need to be equally on top of the mind, to enable clinicians and patients to make the most informed and autonomous decisions about the pain treatment plan formulation as possible. These educational efforts must be consistent in their messaging and aligned with practical clinical practices of primary care frontline practitioners, who are faced with assessing and treating the overwhelming majority of patients with pain and their clinic settings. Clinicians should be instructed about how to be able to distinguish between the patients that can safely be managed with opioid analgesics in their practices, and those patients who would be best managed by a clinician with a higher level of expertise in managing patients with increased risk, such as a pain specialist.

The ability to make educated decisions about whether a consultation or referral to an expert is the best path forward for treating someone with pain is one other aspect of clinician autonomy, and which also needs to be considered. In fact, helping clinicians understand which patients are most appropriate for management in their practice could possibly be one of the most important learnings of all. Complex patients, such as those with a current or preexisting history of substance use, for example, experience pain, and require no less autonomy than other patients do, and it is no less important for clinicians to have the knowledge and sense of autonomy in how these patients are best treated as well. Reproducibly incorporating this information gathering into the pain assessment process could be tremendously valuable for the delivery of consistent pain care with the highest degree of patient autonomy possible.

References

1. Shah P, Thornton I, Turrin D, et al. Informed consent [Updated 2022 Jun 11]. In: StatPearls [Internet]. Treasure Island: StatPearls Publishing; 2023. Available from: https://www.ncbi.nlm.nih.gov/books/NBK430827/. Accessed 27 June 2023.
2. Snyder JE, Gauthier CC. Evidence-Based Medical Ethics: Cases for Practice-Based Learning. Humana Press; 2008. ISBN 978-1-60327-245-2.
3. Dinoff BL. Ethical treatment of people with chronic pain: an application of Kaldjian's framework for shared decision-making. Br J Anaesth. 2019;123(2):e179–82.
4. Scharf A, Voigt L, Vardhana S, Matsoukas K, Wall LM, Arevalo M, Diamond LC. What should clinicians do when a patient's autonomy undermines her being treated equitably? AMA J Ethics. 2021;23(2):E97–108.
5. Drolet BC, White CL. Selective paternalism. Virtual Mentor. 2012;14(7):582–8. https://doi.org/10.1001/virtualmentor.2012.14.7.oped2-1207.
6. Sandman L, Munthe C. Shared decision making, paternalism and patient choice. Health Care Anal. 2010;18(1):60–84.
7. Fernández-Ballesteros R, Sánchez-Izquierdo M, Olmos R, Huici C, Ribera Casado JM, Cruz JA. Paternalism vs. autonomy: are they alternative types of formal care? Front Psychol. 2019;10:1460.
8. Williams GC, Quill TE. Physician autonomy, paternalism, and professionalism: finding our voice amid conflicting duties. Virtual Mentor. 2004;6(2):virtualmentor.2004.6.2.msoc2-0402.
9. Dowell D, Haegerich TM, Chou R. CDC guideline for prescribing opioids for chronic pain – United States, 2016. MMWR Recomm Rep. 2016;65(1):1–49.
10. Lagisetty P, Macleod C, Thomas J, Slat S, Kehne A, Heisler M, Bohnert ASB, Bohnert KM. Assessing reasons for decreased primary care access for individuals on prescribed opioids: an audit study. Pain. 2021;162(5):1379–86.
11. Aviv R. Prescription for disaster: the heartland's pain-pills problem. New Yorker. 2014, April 28.
12. Oliva EM, Bowe T, Manhapra A, Kertesz S, Hah JM, Henderson P, Robinson A, Paik M, Sandbrink F, Gordon AJ, Trafton JA. Associations between stopping prescriptions for opioids, length of opioid treatment, and overdose or suicide deaths in US veterans: observational evaluation. BMJ. 2020;368:m283.
13. Agnoli A, Xing G, Tancredi DJ, Magnan E, Jerant A, Fenton JJ. Association of dose tapering with overdose or mental health crisis among patients prescribed long-term opioids. JAMA. 2021;326(5):411–9.
14. Dowell D, Ragan KR, Jones CM, Baldwin GT, Chou R. CDC clinical practice guideline for prescribing opioids for pain — United States, 2022. MMWR Recomm Rep. 2022;71(RR-3):1–95.
15. 2021 overdose epidemic report: physicians' actions to help end the nation's drug-related overdose and death epidemic —and what still needs to be done. The American Medical Association. https://end-overdose-epidemic.org/. Accessed 15 Nov 2023.
16. Madara JL. The American Medical Association commentary on the CDC 2022 opioid guidelines. Docket no. CDC- 2022-0024.

Beneficence

11

A recurring theme in this book is that the management of pain requires that clinicians apply reproducible approaches with the intention of helping people negotiate pain, suffering, and associated impact on quality of life and function. It is also important that clinicians strive to achieve these goals because of a responsibility to fulfill ethical and moral duties as practitioners and to do so regardless of challenges resulting from external forces which may sometimes be dynamic [1]. As mentioned in the previous chapter, there may be cases where ethical and moral duties involve more than just those that involve the clinician and the patient, considering duties toward the community, and society. It is important to remember that making decisions that are ethically driven by concerns for others does not negatively affect one's ability and duty to provide the most ethical, safe, and effective care to patients.

Beneficence is generally defined as an act of charity, mercy, and kindness, with a sense of duty to promote good, and to act in the best interest of the patient [2, 3]. In the context of general medical and pain care, beneficence can be thought of as the intention to "do good" for patients **in a humanistic fashion**, with professionalism, compassion, and empathy. This ethical principle also incorporates the idea of doing what "is good" for the healthcare professional as well, not referring to economic benefit, but related more to goodness derived from satisfaction and gratification in the delivery of that care. Typically, care which benefits patients with pain often refers to actions which are intended to target the context of the person's pain, their suffering, decreased level of function, and resulting diminished overall quality of life. It is unlikely that "beneficial" pain care could be delivered in the absence of autonomy and shared decision-making, and most often care that benefits the patient does not incorporate a punitive aspects or tonality. It is also unlikely that beneficial pain care could occur in the absence of informed consent as well.

Beneficence in pain care also refers to the delivery of care with a desire to achieve high levels of **communication and understanding**. An important ingredient of beneficent pain care is the identification of mutual patient *and* clinician goals and expectations related to pain treatment. Once identified, these goals and expectations should be discussed in the context of *realism based on the individual patient's*

© The Author(s), under exclusive license to Springer Nature Switzerland AG 2024
K. L. Zacharoff, P. Migdal, *Pain, Drugs, and Ethics*,
https://doi.org/10.1007/978-3-031-63018-7_11

circumstances. Beneficent pain care often *does not* imply eradication of pain, which in many patients with chronic or subacute pain might be unrealistic to expect. But beneficent care does mean that patients and clinicians come to an agreement about what metrics will be utilized to determine progress, lack of progress, or regression. It is also important for patients to understand constraints placed upon clinicians by today's regulatory climate, particularly if a trial of opioid analgesics is considered to be a possible component of a pain treatment plan. This would include the patient understanding what the benefits are of practices which in certain situations might sometimes be perceived as punitive, such as the clinician checking the prescription drug monitoring program database or requesting a specimen for a urine toxicology screen. It is also important to effectively communicate and ensure understanding that **adherence** to a pain treatment plan is a vital aspect of maximizing the potential benefits of pain care. Communication must be easy to understand based on the patient's levels of literacy and numeracy, and avoiding medical jargon, complicated phrases, and unfamiliar terminology.

The relationship between beneficence and "doing no harm" is an intimate one. Although it might seem that by avoiding harm, one is by definition promoting benefit, but that may not necessarily be the case. When managing patients with pain, there is the additional need to consider the fact that the subjective nature of pain symptoms may impact the patient's perspective about perceived benefit. Because of its pervasive use since pain was designated the 5th vital sign, patients might often conclude that a lack in reduction of a pain rating (e.g., numerical pain rating scale 0–10) is insufficient and of no benefit at all. Additionally, as mentioned previously, benefits need to be measured against potential harms to other members of society, especially other members of the patient's household and community members who might gain access to prescribed pain medications, such as opioid analgesics.

Key steps in the delivery of beneficence in pain care are numerous [4]. Emphasis should be placed on **the pain assessment**, which includes capturing **the patient's narrative**, in addition to capturing the standard components of a detailed pain-focused history and physical. Understanding **the patient's individual needs and life impact** are critical pieces of information in helping to determine what course of treatment may be the most beneficial. Additionally, it is important to consider that a humanistic determination of benefit should include not only thinking about pain from a biomedical perspective, but also one that includes a **biopsychosocial perspective** as well. Unique stressors and particular demands that the patient has in addition to their pain symptoms can also be very important factors in helping to identify courses of treatment which may have the most potential benefit. Similar to the importance of adherence, the chance for success of each component of the treatment plan should be considered and individualized as necessary to the patient, and their specific needs. As stated previously, part of the informed consent process involves an analysis of the risks and benefits of each treatment option, and in the case of utilizing controlled substances like opioid analgesics, also needs to consider risks and benefits to others in addition to the patient. An overarching goal should help the patient identify and understand the potential benefit with respect to their overall quality of life instead of just the pain-related symptom(s). Functional capacity should be stressed in this regard as well as a metric of success.

We have already discussed that in some cases, it is not uncommon for a patient to seek pain treatment asking to be told what to do to "make the pain better" in a paternalistic fashion. This may also leave the patient with the impression that engagement, self-management, and active participation are not important components of a pain treatment plan. The opposite is most often true. Beneficence in the context of pain care should also include an assessment of **patient motivation and their willingness to engage**. Passive approaches to treating anything but the most acute instances of pain often have little chance for success and potential benefit in the absence of patient engagement, and the patient acknowledging that they have sense of responsibility that their participation is critical to ensure the highest level of potential benefit. This is just another example of how beneficence is intimately related to informed consent and mutually determined goals and expectations of pain treatment.

Best Interest and Beneficence

In 1910, William J. Mayo [5] stated in his commencement address to the graduating class of Rush Medical College in Chicago that the delivery of healthcare should consider that "**the best interest of the patient is the only interest to be considered**." This simple statement put forth the notion that all discussions about patient care should be able to be distilled down to one driving principle and mandate—that everything healthcare does for patients should be with one goal in mind—that patient needs and their best interests are primary concerns.

It might be reasonable to expect complete alignment with the best interests of the patient and what courses of medical management are most likely going to be beneficial to them, regardless of the best interests of others. But in the case of pain management, that may not necessarily be the case. There can be a variety of stakeholders whose "best interests" might need to be considered with respect to the delivery of pain care. Certainly, **the best interests of the patient** must be primarily considered with respect to delivering **the safest and most effective pain care achievable**.

As mentioned previously, **clinicians may also act in ways that are influenced by what they consider to be their own "best interests,"** which may not be only focused on the best interests of the patient, but also on practicing within local and federal guidelines and mandates in an effort to avoid regulatory scrutiny and possible liability. In some cases, these "interests" have led some clinicians and clinic settings to restrict access to opioid prescriptions in their practices or clinics to serve their own best interests, which may sometimes not coincide with the best interests of the patient, and some situations might be in direct conflict with the patient's best interests. It is not uncommon today for patients in certain clinic settings to be informed that opioid analgesics will not be prescribed under any circumstances, despite the associated consequences of this loss of access to patients, who in some cases might not have anywhere else to seek medical attention. Most of the pain care in the United States is provided to patients by frontline clinicians in primary care settings, such as Family Medicine and Internal Medicine, and it is not surprising that the majority of opioid analgesics have been prescribed by these clinicians in these specialties. If patients are denied access to opioids, even if they might be a potentially appropriate component of treatment, it could become quite difficult for them to find a clinician who would be willing to do so in the absence of a prior clinical relationship. It is also possible that clinicians may not respond positively to being sought out only for the purpose of providing a prescription for an opioid analgesic. One might think that in these situations, a pain specialist might be a viable option, but there are not enough pain specialists or pain clinics to serve the large numbers of pain patients who might be considered to be candidates for pain treatment with opioids, and pain specialists often do not desire to be laden with the sole burden of becoming sources of opioid prescriptions. Another ramification of making a blanket decision to not prescribe opioids under any circumstances may be that when developing a treatment plan, opioids would be by default excluded from the potential treatment options irrespective of their possible value proposition or the patient's risk of portraying aberrant drug-related behaviors.

State medical boards, federal agencies, and other regulators also focus on **the best interests of the household, the community at large, and society**, especially when it comes to issues involving prescribing of controlled substances, such as opioid analgesics and the incidence of overdoses and overdose fatalities. Since the development of the overdose epidemic in our country, virtually every federal and state authority involved in drug approval and regulatory oversight, such as the FDA, the DEA, and the Federation of State Medical Boards, have stressed the importance of considering the risks to people other than the patient when prescribing an opioid analgesic. The mindset of regulators in many cases has shifted away from one with the goal of ensuring access to those people with pain and maintaining the highest possible level of safety and efficacy who may need the prescription medications to one of restricting access and decreasing opioid availability in an effort to serve the best interests of those who may gain access to opioids for nonmedical purposes.

Payers have "best interests" with respect to pain management as well, and in some cases these align with what is most likely to benefit the patient, and in others they may not. Few would dispute the value proposition of a truly multidisciplinary and multimodal approach to managing subacute and chronic pain. Unfortunately, in many cases alternative treatments for pain that are nonopioid and nonpharmacologic may not often be covered by health insurance for a variety of reasons, including cost, evidence basis, or both. This can become quite problematic for patients and clinicians, because in many cases, opioid analgesics are often the least costly option for managing pain and are more often "covered" by insurers than not. Further, newer tamper-resistant formulations of opioids that have been developed to decrease the opioid's risk profile often may not be covered or on formulary because of their increased cost as well.

Other best interest efforts have included finding ways to minimize the variety of different burdens that pain places on our society, irrespective of challenges associated with the overdose epidemic. One example is **the financial burden of pain**. In 2011, the Institute of Medicine Report titled *Relieving Pain in America: A Blueprint for Transforming Prevention, Care, Education, and Research* [6] addressed this issue in detail, estimating that chronic pain alone impacts approximately one-third of the U.S. adult population at any given time, with a financial burden of approximately 565–635 billion dollars annually. This estimate included not only the cost of pain care, but also the costs associated with lost productivity resulting from pain-related decreased functionality and disability. This report also identified several other underlying principles which could be considered to be important factors in considering the best interests of people living in the United States with pain. These included considering that healthcare and its professionals have a moral imperative to provide **effective pain management**, and that it is in the best interests of citizens to consider that imperative as a professional responsibility. This report also stressed that chronic **pain should be considered as a disease itself**; that patients with pain have the right to expect their best interests to be considered in ways similar to those given to people with other medical conditions; that pain treatment should incorporate **not only medical, but also social and psychological approaches** into treatment planning; that **prevention of the development of chronic pain** was as much in the best interests of society as treatment is; that research has been deficient in many respects that it is in the best interest of patients with pain to answer still unanswered questions in order to provide the much needed evidence basis for providing pain care; and that public health approaches which address disparities, stigma, and social determinants of health be considered to be just as important to the best interests of patient care as other important issues.

Best Practices and Beneficence

Traditionally, the development and promulgation of best practices which are clinically relevant to practitioners involved in patient care of a certain medical condition has often resulted in a greater likelihood of a patient's best interests being served, and delivery of care which maximizes both patient and clinician benefit, ultimately yielding overall benefits to society as well. In the context of pain and its management, as stated many other times in this text, there have been numerous practice guidelines, recommendations, and even legislative orders which have intended to achieve the goal of promoting "best practices." In some situations, these efforts have been congruent with each other in some regards, and in other cases, they have been incongruent as well. Dissemination of information regarding these efforts to frontline practitioners has been relatively poor from an educational perspective. Simply mandating education about pain management, for example, does not ensure that the education uniformly adheres to best practices based on current knowledge and desired outcomes. The end result has been a relative **lack of consensus** that has led in many instances to leave clinicians on their own to determine policies and procedures which have the most benefit and also serve patient and societal best interests. It is not difficult to imagine a lack of consistency and congruence when clinicians derive best practices on their own, especially with respect to an often subjective clinical condition like pain.

In 2019, the U.S. Department of Health and Human Services (HHS) published a report titled *Pain Management Best Practices—Interagency Task Force Report* [7] to help provide a basis for consistency and congruence in the delivery of pain care. This comprehensive and well-regarded document was the product of a joint effort of HHS, the U.S. Department of Defense, the U.S. Department of Veterans Affairs, and the White House-based Office of National Drug Control Policy, with the intention of providing clinicians with a resource which considered both goals of acute and chronic pain treatment and the context of the overdose epidemic confronting the United States. One of the key aspects of this report highlighted the intersection of the **best interests** of a patient with pain and delivery of pain **care that is *beneficent***. On the surface, it might seem as if they both refer to the same thing, and in many cases when patients have capacity to make their own medical decisions, they may be identical or closely aligned with each other. However, when helping patients to manage pain, as the intention of the report mentioned above states, **the best interests of the patient *and* societal best interests need to be considered**, without compromising the imperative to deliver beneficent and compassionate care. This report stressed that in order to be beneficial to a patient, pain care must be individualized, and patient-centered. The report continued, stating that with respect to patient's best interests, goals of pain management should focus on measurable improvements, *not* on pain ratings which are completely subjective, but on the **assessment of quality of life, functional capacity**, and the patient's **ability to perform and participate in activities of daily living**. Patients may only expect a reduction in their pain ratings, and there may often be a need to "recalibrate" patient expectations, and educate patients about the potential benefits and their best interests, and consideration of these other metrics as goals of success of pain care.

It is indisputable that opioid anlagesics can provide benefit to a subset of patients suffering from pain, but the question of whether they may or may not serve the patient's (and society's) best interests is a different question. In the context of the abovementioned report and opioid analgesics, there are several recurring themes that are emphasized throughout. First and foremost is the need to identify whether opioid analgesics would be in the best interests of the patient, based on the context of their daily life, the people they have contact with, and the risks associated with potential unhealthy use of prescribed opioids either by the patient or others who might potentially have access to them. A second recurring theme in the HHS report stresses the importance of consistent application of pain treatment approaches and strategies which support both best interests and beneficial care, achieving these goals by a third recurring theme in this report, through education across clinical practices, healthcare professional training programs, and healthcare systems. Lastly, another recurring theme throughout the report worthy of mention is the relationship between patient best interests and insurer reimbursement for the delivery of quality pain care, with equity of access to pain care in order to ensure that all pain treatment options are available to be considered in the development of a mutually determined pain treatment plan with a strong clinician-patient therapeutic alliance.

Clinicians have an ethical responsibility to provide pain care that promotes the patient's well-being and best interests despite the complexities of today's health care system, and without regard to financial or other issues to the greatest degree possible. However, this mandate must carefully balance the well-being, health, and interests of the population at large as well, and never overlooking the needs and best interests of the most vulnerable members of the population who suffer from pain.

References

1. Mark Sullivan MD. Ethical principles in pain management. Pain Med. 2000;1(3):274–9.
2. Kinsinger FS. Beneficence and the professional's moral imperative. J Chiropr Humanit. 2009 Dec;16(1):44–6.
3. Sulmasy LS, Bledsoe TA. ACP ethics, professionalism and human rights committee. American College of Physicians Ethics Manual: seventh edition. Ann Intern Med. 2019;170(2_Suppl):S1–S32.
4. Varkey B. Principles of clinical ethics and their application to practice. Med Princ Pract. 2021;30(1):17–28.
5. Antiel RM, Tilburt JC, Hafferty FW, Brennan MD, Mueller PS. Whose best interest? Minnesota medicine. 2011;94(12):47–9.
6. Institute of Medicine (US). Committee on advancing pain research, care, and education. Relieving pain in America: a blueprint for transforming prevention, care, education, and research. Washington, DC: National Academies Press (US); 2011. PMID: 22553896. ISBN 978-0-309-21484-1
7. U.S. Department of Health and Human Services (2019, May). Pain management best practices inter-agency task force report: updates, gaps, inconsistencies, and recommendations. Retrieved from U. S. Department of Health and Human Services website: https://www.hhs.gov/ash/advisory-committees/pain/reports/index.html. July 3 2023.

Nonmaleficence

12

The omission of an individualized, patient-based ethical analysis as a vital, standard component of pain treatment planning can be just as harmful as utilizing other treatment options which carry risks of harm. It is important to emphasize that pain assessment and treatment planning based on the ethical principles of autonomy, beneficence, nonmaleficence, and justice will often likely involve some blend of all four of these principles, based on the individual patient and their unique life circumstances. This may sometimes necessitate negotiating potential conflicts in the application of these principles, which have the potential to make the process of developing a reproducible ethical approach to pain management somewhat more complex. But it is worth the effort. In fact, in a clinical context, what this translates to is that **developing a process for implementing a reproducible ethical analysis** for the most safe and effective pain treatment plan will best serve clinicians, patients, and their caregivers, and should be part of *all* pain-related assessment and treatment planning. The primary "purpose" of pain treatment is to **alleviate pain and associated suffering to increase overall quality of life and functional capacity to the greatest degree possible in a manner which is as safe and effective as possible.** This is analogous to providing care that is autonomous, equitable, employs informed consent, and shared decision-making considering factors which have a potential to impact adherence, while carefully balancing expected benefits and risks.

Nonmaleficence is the professional ethical obligation of the clinician to not knowingly recommend or employ measures which may cause harm to the patient [1] and is frequently considered by many as *the* "most important ethical edict." "First do no harm" is a universally recognizable phrase used in describing the ethical delivery of health care. Although it is quoted by many to be part of the Hippocratic Oath, in actuality, the phrase "first do no harm" is not specifically mentioned in the Hippocratic Oath. This phrase is from another work by Hippocrates, titled "Of the Epidemics," written in ~400 B.C.E. and translated by Francis Adams in 1849 [Good Press Publishing, 2021].

For clinicians, it is important to remember that there is an intimate relationship between the intent to "do good," recommending measures which will likely benefit

© The Author(s), under exclusive license to Springer Nature Switzerland AG 2024
K. L. Zacharoff, P. Migdal, *Pain, Drugs, and Ethics*,
https://doi.org/10.1007/978-3-031-63018-7_12

the patient most, and the desire to avoid "doing harm" in the management of pain. The desire to help a person who has the capacity to understand risks and benefits associated with possible different courses of pain treatment is critical to this relationship. Virtually every form of medical treatment prescribed to patients in addition to having potential benefit(s) likely also carries some level of risk(s) to the patient, with potential of causing harm. The management of pain is no different. However, there is also often an "elephant in the room," centering around potential harm related to the use of opioid analgesics, even though other medical treatments may carry similar potential for significant harm as well.

Risk, Harm, and Pain Management

Patient-level risk of harm resulting from pain treatment is not a new concept—as mentioned above with respect to other medical treatments, virtually every pain treatment option likely has some potential risks associated with it. It might be natural to, by default, only think about risks associated with opioid analgesics first, but it is important to remember that this applies to other possible components of a pain treatment plan as well. Physical treatments, nonopioid pharmacologic agents, opioid analgesics, interventional treatments, complementary and alternative treatments, and even cognitive behavioral and biopsychosocial approaches carry some degree of risk associated with them. The important step is to assess potential for risk, potential for harm, and potential benefits individually for each patient.

Risk, Harm, and Opioid Analgesics

Specifically with respect to the use of opioid analgesics to treat pain, as with other medications, with potential risk, also comes the potential for harm. Most often, *but not exclusively,* this typically applies to risk and potential harm to the patient. This is where things become a bit interesting with respect to patient-level risk and the potential for harm related to opioid analgesic therapy. In their article titled *Opioid Prescribing and the Ethical Duty to Do No Harm* [2], Nicholson and Hellman stated that from their perspectives as experts in law, clinicians have **two main ethical duties when providing care to people with pain**: first, to **mitigate suffering and cure disease when possible**; and **second, to "do no harm."** They further state that **clinicians have a duty to adhere to these two directives because of their responsibility to the patient**, while **regulators are responsible for having a duty to protect members of society from harm.** They proposed that clinicians should not necessarily have to consider potential societal harms when making decisions about benefit and harm to individuals, especially in the context of the utilization of opioid analgesics as a component of a pain treatment plan when determined to be appropriate for the patient. Additionally, the authors emphasized that clinicians are bound to similar ethical duties to those patients already being prescribed opioids for their pain.

The abovementioned article is just one illustration of some of the controversies clinicians who treat patients with pain with opioid analgesics and regulators who govern their use face today. Regulators such as the U.S. Food and Drug Administration (FDA) are tasked with protecting patients from harm by ensuring that the drug approval process is primarily purposed with the goal of ensuring safety and efficacy of a given medication or treatment modality if used in the context and indications for which its use is being proposed. But it is important to underscore that this in no way guarantees that if an FDA-approved medication is used for a different purpose (i.e., "off-label) that it will be safe and efficacious in those circumstances. That has typically been left to the discretion of the prescribing clinician in the past, and continues to be so today. In simpler terms, this means that the FDA does not consider, or even need to consider, all possible uses of a medication as part of its drug approval process, just some reasonable representative scientifically verified samples of demonstration of safety, efficacy, and potential of risk and harm. While this means that the FDA restricts a pharmaceutical manufacturer from commercially advertising and promoting off-label prescribing and use of a medication, clinicians are free to make shared decisions with patients about this type of use at will without ethical compromise. This includes the use of opioid analgesics in clinical practice. In fact, the FDA has little to no authority over clinician prescribing patterns and the clinical use of approved medications.

However, the FDA *does* have the ability to incorporate certain types of requirements to enhance safety and minimize risk into the drug approval process, and the post-approval use of medications as well. One mechanism that the FDA frequently uses to mitigate risk is the requirement that a drug have a **REMS, or Risk Evaluation and Mitigation Strategy**. The authority to require a REMS for a particular drug or class of drugs was given to the FDA in 2007 by the FDA Amendments Act (Section 505-1), with the intention of giving the FDA a mechanism of ensuring that the benefits of a drug outweigh its risks beyond its labeling. If the FDA decides that a REMS is necessary, several components may be included. For example, a medication guide or package insert that is patient-friendly (with respect to literacy) and easy to understand may be required. Additionally, a specific communication plan about risks and benefits might need to be sent to all healthcare professionals who are potential prescribers. Other specific elements to ensure safe use may also be required, such as specialized education and certification of prescribers and possibly also dispensers (e.g., pharmacy staff), restriction to using the medication in certain specific clinical settings for use and administration (e.g., hospitals), and a requirement that the pharmaceutical manufacturer(s) supply the FDA with a detailed plan of implementation of any required safety strategies.

One well-known example of an FDA-required REMS is associated with a drug named isotretinoin, a prescription medication used for the treatment of acne (Accutane®) that has been shown to be associated with increased risk of teratogenicity in children related to fetal exposure. This is an example of an FDA-approved medication which has a certain risk profile, has been shown to have significant efficacy, but also carries with it significant risk. The same situation applies to opioid analgesics. In July 2012, the FDA made the decision (considering the public health risks associated with opioid prescribing and unintended overdoses and overdose fatalities) to require a REMS for extended-release/long-acting opioid analgesics [3] (ER/LA opioid analgesics). According to the FDA, the decision to limit the REMS to just ER/LA formulations of opioids at that time was to gauge the logistic viability of such a program for such a very commonly prescribed class of medications. The rationale was that while ER/LA opioid analgesics offered significant potential patient benefits, including convenience (e.g., less frequent dosing), they also carried a degree of increased risk because each pill had a higher and potentially more dangerous amount of opioid in it. The hallmark of the ER/LA opioid REMS was that it applied to *all* ER/LA opioids and their manufacturers (brand name and generic), making it what was referred to as a "class-wide" REMS. One major element of the ER/LA REMS was to ensure safe use by the implementation of a prescriber education program covering the general risks of opioid medications, in addition to safe prescribing practices and safe use by patients. ER/LA opioid manufacturers were required to collectively fund the development of the educational programs, dissemination, administration of them, and to conduct and report an analysis of their successful deployment and effectiveness to the FDA. In 2018, considering the increasing numbers of opioid-related overdoses in the United States, the FDA expanded the opioid REMS to include immediate-release/short-acting (IR/SA) opioid analgesics as well. Once again, the impetus was to ensure that the benefits of opioid analgesic use outweighed the potential risks of harm.

It is important to note that the implementation the abovementioned educational elements of the opioid REMS to assure safe use, clinician were (and are) *voluntary* educational activities. At the time of the opioid REMS implementation, the FDA did not and still does not have the authority to require prescribers to participate in educational programs that do not require some type of certification, such as the abovementioned isotretinoin REMS, which precludes "uncertified" (clinicians who have fulfilled the educational requirement) clinicians from prescribing it.

The regulatory agency that *does* have the authority to effect change in clinician prescribing patterns of controlled substances like opioid analgesics to prevent patient harm is the **Drug Enforcement Administration (DEA)**. The DEA is the federal agency that most directly has the authority to oversee access to controlled substances, the ability to regulate (and limit) the manufacturing and distribution of controlled substances, such as opioid analgesics, and to investigate and prosecute individuals who are supsected to have acted unlawfully in prescribing or diverting controlled substances or distributing illicit drugs (e.g., heroin, fentanyl, etc.). The DEA manages a healthcare professional's ability to prescribe controlled substances by requiring registration for that "privilege," and monitors data from many different sources, including the state-managed prescription drug monitoring databases (PDMPs) to identify prescribing patterns which may be suspicious and worthy of investigation. In addition to several other tactics at its disposal, the DEA (unlike the FDA) does have the ability to require mandatory educational programs for prescribers as deemed necessary with the intention of **protecting members of society from harm.**

Since 2010, when the "opioid epidemic" in the United States was first formally identified, there has been some "blurring of the lines" between a clinician's responsibility to treat patients with pain if opioids were deemed appropriate, and regulatory actions to opioid prescribing in order to protect the public at large. The seemingly ever-increasing number of opioid-related deaths has continued to frustrated legislators and regulators who collectively decided that what needed to happen to curb drug-associated loss of life was tighter regulation of their use, increased scrutiny of clinicians who "over-relied" on utilizing opioids to treat patients with pain, and ultimately a decrease in the number of opioid prescriptions and dosage and quantity prescribed. Additionally, and very much related to the 2016 CDC opioid guidelines, the collective regulatory mindset was that for patients who were being prescribed chronic opioid therapy in large quantities and/or higher dosages, that **de-prescribing, or tapering** pain patients who were being treated with opioids on a chronic basis was another important strategy in helping to mitigate the risk of opioid-related overdose and overdose fatalities. All of this with the intention of preventing harm not only to patients, but members of the community and society. What may not have been foreseen was the potential for harm that might result from these efforts. It is also possible that the "risk" of causing harm from forced tapering of opioids and de-prescribing them to patients in need might not have been considered to be important. In fact, trends that illustrate the potential for harm associated with tapering or stopping opioids are starting to appear in scientific literature. One retrospective analysis in the U.S. VA Health System examined the association of stopping opioids and overdose or suicide-related deaths [4] and found that 57.4% of 2887 deaths from overdose and suicide in a one-year period involved patients for whom opioids were discontinued after being component of the pain treatment plan. Another retrospective analysis of 113,618 patients [5] found that "among patients prescribed stable long-term, higher dose opioid therapy, tapering events actually were significantly associated with *increased* risk of overdose and mental health crisis."

There has been significant debate for and against the therapeutic value proposition of utilizing opioid analgesics to treat pain in both short- and long-term situations. Those arguing against claim that in many cases, pain can be safely and adequately managed with other modalities, including nonopioid analgesics, avoiding the potential opioid risks associated with aberrant behaviors and the potential for addiction. What is often missing from those arguing *against* the use of opioids is the consideration of weighing the risk of harm associated with the use of those pharmacologic alternatives such as NSAIDs or acetaminophen (discussed later in this chapter) compared to those associated with opioids. Alternatively, many also reference a lack of scientific evidence demonstrating a long-term benefit in terms of pain treatment outcomes, including improved quality of life and function for patients prescribed long-term opioid therapy. Those arguing *for* the use of opioid therapy cite many instances where opioids have been a "life preserver" for people, who would suffer tremendously if denied opioids as part of their pain treatment plan. There has also been a public outcry from chronic pain patients being treated with opioids that, in some cases, they have been finding increasingly difficult to find clinicians willing to prescribe them, despite their demonstrated value in maintaining quality of life and enabling a higher level of function in the face of pain. Social media shows a significant decrease in patient satisfaction and decreased efficacy of pain management in both acute and chronic situations due to the desire to avoid prescribing or to discontinue opioids at all costs by many healthcare professionals as a result of negative regulatory and mainstream media messaging about them.

From an ethical perspective, it seems that the duty to avoid harm and consider the risks and benefits associated with all treatment options comparatively may be taking a bit of a back seat to the debate about the pros and cons of opioid prescribing itself. **Tolerance to opioids**, for example, is often cited as an adverse effect or aberrant phenomenon by many who argue against opioid use, when, in virtually all cases (depending on specific metabolic pathways), tolerance is actually a normal state of physiologic adaptation, and while it does pose a risk due to a need for increased dosing to achieve analgesic effect, it does not by default lead to harm as long as it is expected and clinically managed accordingly. Additionally, there may sometimes be a lack of clarity and consensus with respect to the differences between dependence on opioids and addiction to opioids, with these two terms often being used interchangeably with each other as if they were synonomous. This lack of clarity has in many cases left clinicians unable to discern between the risks of deprescribing or tapering of opioids and risks associated with their continuation.

To clarify some of the potential harms associated with blanket dose reduction and discontinuation of long-term opioid analgesic therapy, the Department of Health and Human Services (HHS) issued a guidance for clinicians on this topic titled "*HHS Guide for Clinicians on the Appropriate Dosage Reduction or Discontinuation of Long-Term Opioid Analgesics*" in 2019 [6]. In this guide, the HHS stressed the fact that while more "judicious use" of opioid analgesics has the potential to benefit patients as well as public health, there should still be consideration whether the benefits outweigh the risks associated with their use. Additionally, this guidance also emphasized that because of the potential for harm, opioids should be prescribed in a manner that is "thoughtful, deliberative, collaborative, and measured," considering "the individual patient's diagnosis, circumstances, and unique needs." This guidance specifically identified examples of situations where the avoidance of harm warranted discontinuation or tapering, including improvement in pain (including QOL and functional capacity), the patient requesting the desire to do so, a need for opioid dosage increases in the absence of clinical progress, evidence of aberrant behaviors (e.g., unhealthy use), adverse effects, an overdose, identifying that the patient is receiving a concurrent prescription for benzodiazepines, the patient has comorbid medical conditions which increase the potential for harm, or long-term opioid therapy in the absence of a determination of a *current* benefit/harm analysis.

This HHS guidance also identified situations **where the decision to taper or discontinue opioid may pose risks as well**. These include: **insistance on tapering or discontinuation** by the clinician even when the benefits of continuing opioid therapy outweigh the risks, **misinterpreting cautionary dosing thresholds** as "mandates" for clinical care without considering individual patient situations, **not considering the fact that there are patients who may be co-prescribed opioids and benzodiazepines for valid medical reasons**, **threatening to "fire" patients who are unwilling to agree to discontinuation or tapering**, and a **lack of consideration of the risks associated with withdrawal when tapering in physically**

dependent patients, as well as **risks of increased pain, anxiety, depression, suicidal ideation, self-harm, diminished trust, and opioid seeking from illicit sources**.

Lastly, the HHS guidance emphasizes the importance of shared decision-making about the possible utility of opioid analgesics with patients, helping them to determine the best course of action in the context of their unique life circumstances. Unfortunately, as described in many other parts of this book, dissemination of the HHS guidance to those in clinical practice in concert with education has been lacking or completely absent, with clinicians being much more aware of "regulatory risk" instead of patient benefit and avoidance of harm related to *all* possible courses of action in a pain treatment plan.

Risk, Harm, and Nonopioid Medications

For many years, **nonsteroidal anti-inflammatory drugs (NSAIDs) have been recognized to carry a significant adverse effect profile**, with some estimates in the past suggesting that more than 100,000 patients are hospitalized each year because of NSAID-related complications, and approximately 16,500 patients dying annually of NSAID-related complications, resulting in an economic burden of at least $4 billion per year in the United States [7]. As increased cardiovascular risk of NSAIDs has come to be recognized in the geriatric patient population (those over age 65), more attention started to focus on minimizing harm related to this class of medications, especially given the increased rate of arthritis-related pain, degenerative spine conditions, and other pain-causing conditions in this patient population [8]. In fact, the 2009 revision of pain management guidelines in older adults recommended that considering the potential for gastrointestinal and cardiovascular risk of harm associated with NSAIDs, these drugs should be used "rarely or with extreme caution" in older patients. Additionally, as new evidence began to develop with respect to the increased cardiovascular risks associated with NSAIDs, in many cases they were considered to be relatively contraindicated in patients with a prior history of a variety of preexisting medical conditions including cardiovascular disease, hypertension, and renal disease [9].

Despite these concerns, and likely related to both their availability over the counter, their anti-inflammatory properties, and their nonaddictive nature, NSAIDs have come to occupy a prominent role as opioid alternatives, and they are among the most widely prescribed medications in the United States today. In fact, considering the regulatory movement toward more restrictive prescribing of opioid analgesics because of their role in the overdose epidemic, NSAIDs have been recommended by many opioid prescribing guidelines as "safer" and, in many cases, equally effective, nonopioid pharmacologic pain treatments.

The ethical challenge for clinicians with respect to NSAIDs is balancing patient-level benefit and risk of harm compared to opioid analgesics. From a regulatory perspective, there is a clear desire to emphasize and increase the utility of NSAIDs at least as first-line analgesic medications because of community and societal risks related to opioid prescriptions, and their speculated role in fueling the overdose crisis. Another dimension of ethical challenge is clinician fear of retribution for what regulators identify as "overprescribing" or "inappropriately" prescribing opioids which in many cases may not be deemed by the regulators to be "necessary," when nonopioids such as NSAIDs could have been employed.

Another frequently considered nonopioid analgesic pharmacologic alternative is **acetaminophen**. In fact, acetaminophen is the first recommended medication for pain treatment in the World Health Organization's "analgesic ladder" [10]. Although its specific mechanism of action is postulated and widely debated, acetaminophen *is* something which should be considered as a first-line, nonopioid analgesic agent in patients who have a relative or absolute contraindication for NSAID use, such as patients at an advanced age (over the age of 65), relevant gastrointestinal history, cardiovascular history, or a history of renal disease. However, like NSAIDs, **acetaminophen has a significant risk profile as well,** especially with respect to its deleterious effects on the liver. Acute liver failure is defined as a severe hepatic dysfunction, usually in people without a prior history of liver disease. While infectious hepatitis is the most common cause of acute liver failure, drug-induced hepatitis with ensuing liver failure accounts for nearly half of the cases of acute liver failure in the United States, with **acetaminophen toxicity being the most common cause** [11]. Additionally, it is thought that in terms of long-term analgesic use, acetaminophen may be less valuable than previously thought [12]. It has been well recognized that therapeutic doses of acetaminophen have been associated with increased levels of liver markers indicative of hepatic injury, although subclinical in nature. Some research points toward a link between chronic ingestion of acetaminophen and liver damage. In the context of potential harm, there seems to be increasing evidence that the long-term use of acetaminophen for chronic pain is associated with significant adverse effects, which may or may not be serious in nature. It has been referred by some to be a "least-worst" first-line pain treatment option for chronic pain [12].

An average pharmacy in the United States has approximately 200 or more products which are available over the counter that contain acetaminophen. Inadvertent overdose of acetaminophen may result from analgesic use and unintentional co-administration of other products which are available over the counter that also contain acetaminophen. This risk is real and is one of the reasons that patients should be informed that self-administration of acetaminophen for longer than three days should include contacting a healthcare professional to try to mitigate this potential risk. It may not be apparent to most patients that these products contain acetaminophen and present these potential risks.

Patients with a history of liver disease are not likely to be good candidates for acute or chronic pain treatment with acetaminophen. It is also possible that patients with liver disease may also have other comorbid medical conditions which might preclude them from being appropriate candidates for treatment with an NSAID as well. It is also possible in these patients that opioid analgesics might be safer pain treatment options in these patient populations.

Adherence, Risk, and Harm

Part of a clinician's role in the ethical principle of "doing no harm" is to gauge the likelihood of a patient adhering to a treatment plan. While it might not seem apparent, **a lack of patient adherence** to a mutually developed pain treatment plan can in certain circumstances carry just as much risk as other treatment options, and from an ethical perspective it needs to be considered. Patient nonadherence may be determined to be intentional, unintentional, or some combination of both.

There are a multitude of factors which can play a role in driving nonadherence. **From the patient perspective**, **behavioral factors** may impact adherence, such as prior/baseline levels of physical activity, health-related interests, motivation, and willingness to invest financially in their treatment. Fear, anxiety, cognitive capacity, cues from others, and even self-image can also negatively impact patient adherence to a pain treatment plan [13]. **Nonbehavioral patient factors** can contribute to nonadherence as well, such as including patient demographics, household stability, socio-economic status, level of mobility, and level of education. A patient's prior history with pain may also potentially impact the likelihood of adherence if their past experiences with pain treatment have been negative ones. Additionally, **the presence of other comorbid medical conditions** might sometimes present too much of a challenge for patients to deal with, which may result in conceding that pain is part of their life and not as important as managing their other medical conditions and treatments. It is not uncommon for patients to be less likely to adhere to a treatment plan i**f they have seen multiple healthcare providers for the same pain-related complaint**—patients may lose faith, and just "go through the motions" for a variety of reasons, lacking confidence which may cause them to not adhere to the treatment plan. Alternatively, patients who have seen many other providers for the same pain complaint **may have had negative experiences with certain treatments** (e.g., adverse effects), and be less likely to follow prescribed treatments because they have negative expectations.

From the clinic/clinician perspective, **clinical expertise in pain management and the clinician/clinic consensus on how pain should best be managed** may sometimes lead to mixed messaging to the patient and nonadherence to a pain treatment plan, especially if there are differences in viewpoints about the most appropriate treatment choices (e.g., opioid analgesic therapy). **A clinician's prior experiences** with treating certain patients with pain could also lead to precognitive judgment about expectations of patient adherence which may then be transferred to the patient, potentially negatively influencing likelihood of adherence, and ultimately chances for successful treatment.

Both clinician and patient beliefs and attitudes about pain treatments may influence the likelihood of adherence and treatment outcomes [14]. For example, concerns about dependence, development of adverse effects, and tolerance may lead to the clinician and/or the patient to put little faith in the chance of success, and the risk/benefit profile, leading to a de facto mistrust in the treatment plan with the potential for a low level of adherence to it. Research has shown that when clinician endorsement of mutually determined pain treatment options is positive, patient adherence is likely to be increased [15].

There *are* critical components of adherence to pain treatment which can maximize benefit and minimize harm [15], the most important being **effective communication between the clinician and patient**. Patients need to understand the significance of self-management as a component of pain treatment, and that they have responsibilities in mitigating risk and maximizing efficacy. Patient-centric care that considers and incorporates patient needs based individual differences in the patient's prior experiences, priorities, and viewpoints are more likely to benefit than harm the patient. Further, patient education about their pain-related diagnosis can have a significant impact on fostering adherence and mitigating risk associated with nonadherence.

Harm Reduction, Risk, and Harm

Sometimes the term "**harm reduction**" in the context of opioid analgesics refers to the same thing as the employment of the ethical principle of nonmaleficence when assessing and attempting to reduce risk of opioid therapy as a component of a pain treatment plan. The **Substance Abuse and Mental Health Services Administration (SAMHSA)** defines "harm reduction" as a set of strategies to help stem the "most significant substance use and overdose epidemic the United States has ever faced [16]." This includes an emphasis specifically on prevention of opioid overdose and opioid overdose-related fatalities, infectious disease transmission associated with unhealthy drug use, improving the biopsychosocial well-being of people who use drugs such as opioids for nonmedical purposes, and offering increased access to "low-threshold" options for opioid use disorder treatment and other related care. **In simpler terms, "harm reduction" in this context refers to saving lives.**

In many situations, harm reduction does not refer to improving the lives of patients with pain, but to saving the lives of others (i.e., not the patient). In addition to the abovementioned intentions of harm reduction strategies, decreased or optimized opioid prescribing has been included by many regulators and guidelines as a key component of any opioid-related harm reduction. But there is growing concern about misinterpretation of this specific strategy in that it may result in an imbalance between the desired goals of saving the lives of people with addiction and potential risk of overdose and delivering safe and effective pain care to patients in need of pain relief, sometimes resulting in harm to patients who may be appropriate candidates for opioid analgesic therapy [17]. Another important concern related to harm is a growing sense that patients with chronic pain who might be potential candidates for opioid therapy have concerns about becoming targets of stigmatization. Potential harm to clinicians can occur if they fear being stigmatized and labeled as "over-prescribers" of opioids, regardless of the intended clinical rationale. In either case, stigma has the potential to cause "harm" by creating barriers to access to care for patients with pain, which has the potential to cause significant harm.

A recurring theme throughout this book involves education, underscoring that **education can be one of the most important strategies with respect to achieving "harm reduction,"** with its primary mission being to help identify the intersection of reducing harm to patients for whom pain treatment with opioid analgesic may be appropriate and mitigating the potential for risk of aberrant behaviors, addiction, overdose/overdose fatality, and appropriately navigating that intersection. The relationship between pain treatment with opioids and the overdose epidemic is unquestionably a complex one, but this does not mean that it is impossible to reduce harm if they are deemed necessary. Simple steps can be taken and have been recommended to help achieve these goals, including simply asking patients about their past or present history or substance use, as well as substance use history of other members of the immediate household. Warning patients about safe storage of opioids is a critical harm reduction strategy, and requires communicating an appropriate sense of responsibility to patients about their role in preventing harm to others who may have access and intentionally or unintentionally suffer negative consequences as a result of access to them. Speaking to patients about the importance of disposing of opioids (and how that should be accomplished) when they are no longer needed is another important step in preventing harm because a significant number of illicit substance users report that they began using opioids that were originally prescribed to others, or obtained from a family member or friend. Educating patients about the fact that sharing a prescribed controlled substance like an opioid with anyone else is against the law everywhere in the United States, and that they may have liability if they share it with someone, and that person suffers harm as a result. Another not well-disseminated but important but relatively simple harm reduction strategy was recommended in 2020, when the **United States Preventive Services Task Force recommended screening _all_ adults 18 years of age and older for unhealthy drug use** [18] by asking the patient questions about it, as opposed to testing biological specimens (e.g., urine toxicology screening), with the intention that it could help prevent harm by identifying patients at risk and factoring that information into the risk/benefit analysis and offering them resources about treatment for unhealthy drug use.

It is important to consider that "harm reduction" does not need to be pain treatment reduction or discontinuation, and that primary prevention is not the same thing as denying appropriate patients in need access to pain medications or other pain treatments.

References

1. Varkey B. Principles of clinical ethics and their application to practice. Med Princ Pract. 2021;30(1):17–28.
2. Nicholson KM, Hellman D. Opioid prescribing and the ethical duty to do no harm. Am J Law Med. 2020;46(2-3):297–310.
3. American Council for Continuing Medical Education. CME for FDA REMS. https://www.accme.org/cme-for-fda-rems. Accessed 6 July 2023.

4. Oliva EM, Bowe T, Manhapra A, Kertesz S, Hah JM, Henderson P, Robinson A, Paik M, Sandbrink F, Gordon AJ, Trafton JA. Associations between stopping prescriptions for opioids, length of opioid treatment, and overdose or suicide deaths in US veterans: observational evaluation. BMJ. 2020;368:m283.

5. Agnoli A, Xing G, Tancredi DJ, Magnan E, Jerant A, Fenton JJ. Association of dose tapering with overdose or mental health crisis among patients prescribed long-term opioids. JAMA. 2021;326(5):411–9. https://doi.org/10.1001/jama.2021.11013. Erratum in: JAMA. 2022 Feb 15;327(7):688. Erratum in: JAMA. 2022 Feb 15;327(7):687

6. National Institute on Drug Abuse. HHS guide for clinicians on the appropriate dosage reduction or discontinuation of long-term opioid analgesics. https://nida.nih.gov/nidamed-medical-health-professionals/opioid-crisis-pain-management/hhs-guide-clinicians-appropriate-dosage-reduction-or-discontinuation-long-term-opioid. Accessed 7 July 2023.

7. Fine M. Quantifying the impact of NSAID-associated adverse events. Am J Manag Care. 2013;19(14 Suppl):s267–72.

8. Kuehn BM. New pain guideline for older patients: avoid NSAIDs, consider opioids. JAMA. 2009;302(1):19.

9. Varga Z, Sabzwari SRA, Vargova V. Cardiovascular risk of nonsteroidal anti-inflammatory drugs: an under-recognized public health issue. Cureus. 2017;9(4):e1144.

10. Anekar AA, Hendrix JM, Cascella M. WHO analgesic ladder. [Updated 2023 Apr 23]. In: StatPearls [Internet]. Treasure Island (FL): StatPearls Publishing; 2024 Jan-. Available from: https://www.ncbi.nlm.nih.gov/books/NBK554435/.

11. Shah NJ, Royer A, John S. Acute liver failure. [Updated 2022 Jul 18]. In: StatPearls [Internet]. Treasure Island (FL): StatPearls Publishing; 2022 Jan-. Available from: https://www.ncbi.nlm.nih.gov/books/NBK482374/. Accessed 7 July 2023.

12. McCrae JC, Morrison EE, MacIntyre IM, Dear JW, Webb DJ. Long-term adverse effects of paracetamol – a review. Br J Clin Pharmacol. 2018;84(10):2218–30.

13. Wilson PR. Facilitating treatment adherence in pain medicine. Pain Med. 2018;19(6):1290–2.

14. Timmerman L, Stronks DL, Huygen FJ. The relation between patients' beliefs about pain medication, medication adherence, and treatment outcome in chronic pain patients: a prospective study. Clin J Pain. 2019;35(12):941–7.

15. Butow P, Sharpe L. The impact of communication on adherence in pain management. Pain. 2013;154(Suppl 1):S101–7.

16. SAMHSA. Harm reduction. https://www.samhsa.gov/find-help/harm-reduction. Accessed 7 July 2023.

17. Wade CL, Goracke-Postle CJ. Harm reduction strategies for chronic pain management in the opioid epidemic. R Street Policy Study No. 142, May 2018.

18. US Preventive Services Task Force, Krist AH, Davidson KW, Mangione CM, Barry MJ, Cabana M, Caughey AB, Curry SJ, Donahue K, Doubeni CA, Epling JW Jr, Kubik M, Ogedegbe G, Pbert L, Silverstein M, Simon MA, Tseng CW, Wong JB. Screening for unhealthy drug use: US preventive services task force recommendation statement. JAMA. 2020;323(22):2301–9.

Justice

13

It might be natural to think of justice in healthcare in a purely legal sense, relating to things such as the administration of law(s), law enforcement, and maintaining a state of lawful behavior—in other words, a right to be protected. As an ethical principle in healthcare, justice has a somewhat different meaning, more related to fairness of access, equity in assessment and treatment, and fair and equitable distribution of available resources. It can then be extrapolated that from a healthcare perspective, justice refers to rights. Rights include having access, a right to be treated equitably, and the right to not be a victim of discrimination. Many consider that it is a patient's fundamental human right to have their pain assessed and treated adequately [1], treated no differently than patients with other medical conditions, and utilizing all available options for treatment possible without discrimination. In the context of managing pain, "patient need" can be impacted by several factors, including the potential for a certain treatment or components of a treatment plan to ultimately benefit the patient, the urgency of pain relief to alleviate suffering, the potential for a pain treatment to positively impact the patient's quality of life, and the degree of durability of the potential benefit(s) that pain treatment may have. Alternatively, many have also debated whether or not the "right to pain treatment" is more of a legal construct requiring legislation to enable its enforcement as a "right" or if it is purely an ethical term, defining and underscoring a healthcare professional's ethical and moral duty to relieve a patient's pain and suffering whenever possible within the confines of the law and accepted clinical practice(s).

Justice is an ethical principle that is sometimes not as clear-cut as autonomy, beneficence, and nonmaleficence. In the context of pain management, justice means much more than just having the right to be treated for pain and associated suffering. Justice means that people with pain have **a right to be** *respected*. Justice means that people with pain have **a right to be treated** *with dignity*. Justice means that people with pain have **a right to be treated and** *informed truthfully*. Justice means that people have **the right to** *be believed*.

Justice is commonly defined in terms of fairness, moral correctness, and a healthcare system where every person is entitled to the same benefits and treatment from that

© The Author(s), under exclusive license to Springer Nature Switzerland AG 2024

K. L. Zacharoff, P. Migdal, *Pain, Drugs, and Ethics*,

https://doi.org/10.1007/978-3-031-63018-7_13

system, including rights which are inherent or natural and **within the confines of the law(s)** as it/they apply. Elements of justice include ensuring **access to resources, equity in treatment, consideration of diversity, participation in the development of policies, defining rights which are afforded just by being human**, applying to all individuals in given society. Sometimes, justice may be confused with autonomy, which refers to the right for **an individual** with capacity to direct the healthcare they receive. Two common classifications of justice as an ethical principle in healthcare are distributive justice and social justice. **Distributive justice** refers to an ethical duty to deliver care fairly and equitably for patients in need [2]. **Social justice** refers to the idea that everyone has the right to expect that the medical care they are offered and receive is equal to that offered to others regardless of race, gender, religion, or any other attribute.

Patient Rights

Few would argue that the need for, and right to adequate pain care is less important today than it was in 2000, when pain was designated the 5th vital sign, but as mentioned elsewhere in this text, polarization about pain and its treatment in the medical, political, regulatory, and patient communities is *real*. It is not uncommon today to read about clinicians who have considered the best course of action to be to steer clear of caring for patients with pain as their "safest" course of action for a variety of reasons, including fear of regulatory scrutiny, negative media attention, and possible labeling as "over-prescribers" if opioid analgesics were considered to be used. It is important to note that along with designating pain as a "vital sign," a *Pain Patient Bill of Rights* [3] was created as well, with the "rights" listed as:

- The right to be cared for by the healthcare professional of the patient's choice
- The right to ask questions about a clinician's education, licensure, and clinical experience
- The right to pain care that is respectful, objective, and non-discriminatory
- The right to have pain managed safely and effectively
- The right to ask for and receive a referral to a specialist
- The right to have examinations regularly and to have the pain treatment plan continued or adjusted based on goals and expectations
- The right to receive understandable information related to risks and benefits of all pain treatment options
- The right to refuse suggested treatment options
- The right to a second opinion with respect to diagnosis and treatment
- The right to participate in their pain treatment decisions, and if the patient lacks capacity
- The right to be represented by designated family members and/or guardians
- Rights related to access of medical records, costs associated with treatment, confidentiality, and the complaint and appeals processes.

Along the spectrum of the intersection of pain, drugs, and ethics, it should be noted that despite the notion that an evidence basis should always be the foundation of good medical practice, in many situations the treatment of pain is often considered to be "neither an absolute science nor risk-free [4]." It is unquestionable that with pain being one of the single most common reasons that people seek medical attention that the lion's share of managing patients with pain often falls on the shoulders of frontline clinicians in the Primary Care setting. If frontline practitioners continue to step away from caring for patients with pain, then in many cases, patients may be left with nowhere to turn to seek pain treatment due to the relatively small number of pain specialists relative to the large number of people in the United States with pain. This could be thought of as an *injustice,* if indeed all patients do actually have a "right" to receive pain care.

In 2007, Fishman [4] referred to pain medicine as "an orphan" in general medical practices, often making it difficult to support the case for identifying the assessment and treatment of pain as a basic human right, and in some cases even leading to further conflict about pain treatment as a priority in medicine and medical ethics from the perspective of justice. Fishman also postulated that how pain management was positioned and integrated throughout healthcare in the future could significantly impact how medicine defines and meets its obligations to people with pain, and in the absence of major changes in medical education, research, and clinical care. Fishman also foreshadowed that the U.S. society at large would be faced with dealing with challenges related to conflicting priorities of policies, legislation, and litigation related to aberrant drug use, addiction, overdose fatalities, and public safety, along with the potential for unintended negative consequences regarding the rights of people with pain and those who treat it.

To date, not much has changed with respect to justice and the right to have pain adequately assessed and treated since Fishman's article in 2007, and in some ways things have deteriorated with respect to pain treatment, including poorer pain treatment for disparate patient populations, and a lack of coordinated efforts to better educate clinicians in practice, future clinicians, patients, and caregivers. Logistical barriers that increasingly deny access to patients in need and the implementation of regulatory and political tactics and strategies may also be having unintended negative consequences on access to pain care. It is not uncommon today to see research which demonstrates that pain continues to be inadequately addressed. This is despite the fact that it is well substantiated that the undertreatment of pain can result in patients with pain unjustly suffering not only physically, but also psychologically, socially, and in many cases economically. There is also a significant cost and added financial burden to society not only from the increased cost of care and utilization of resources (such as Emergency Department visits) for people with poorly or undertreated pain, but also resulting from lost productivity resulting from both **absenteeism** and **presenteeism** (being present at work with pain, with diminished efficiency or capacity).

The Department of Health and Human Services 2019 *Pain Management Best Practices Inter-Agency Task Force Report* [5] outlined a number of steps which could be taken to correct deficiencies identified and help to fulfill the mandate that every person is entitled to be provided safe and effective pain care fairly and equitably. These include **increasing the dissemination *and* use of congruent and**

coordinated clinical practice guidelines in clinical practice settings and health-care systems which not only focus on mitigating the overdose epidemic, but also **focusing on consistently improving the quality of pain care**, with the goals of improving quality of life, functionality, and the ability to better perform activities of daily living. Additionally, this report emphasized the importance of alleviating suffering by addressing associated barriers to care including stigma, lack of access to care, and issues related to insurance coverage (or lack of it) and reimbursement policies for all possible pain treatment options.

Dignity and Justice

As an ethical principle, **justice also affords patients with pain, their families, and their caregivers the right to expect to be treated with dignity** [6]. In addition to the traditional ethical mandates of autonomy, beneficence, nonmaleficence, and justice, treating patients with dignity incorporates consideration of factors more than solely risks and benefits, often including **their emotional state**, **relationships with others**, **goals and expectations of pain treatment**, **desire for privacy**, and **beliefs** about the sanctity of their body and ability to make decisions related to that sanctity. From a clinical perspective, the intersection of caring, justice, and dignity is the practice of pain care with high levels of communication, compassion, empathy, and realism. From a patient perspective, the intersection of caring, justice, and dignity includes consideration of input from family members and other decision makers with the same level of respect afforded to the patient, especially in situations where the capacity of the patient to make their own medical decisions is waning or absent (e.g., dementia).

Pain, Individual Justice, and Societal Justice

As mentioned earlier in this chapter and elsewhere in this text, clinicians are encouraged to utilize the ethical principles for the purpose of providing an ability to deliver ethically appropriate care by incorporating reproducible approaches into the analysis of risk, benefit, harm, communication, and comprehension. Most common medical conditions dictate an ethical imperative to consider **patient-level risk and patient-level benefit**, based on the right for patients to be offered options for treatment which balance patient-level safety with patient-level efficacy. Sometimes, societal justice and individual justice don't necessarily coincide with each other. Sometimes, the needs of "the many" may outweigh the needs of "the few."

The evolution of the overdose epidemic facing our country and its relationship with opioid analgesics has dictated the need for a different ethical equation and analysis with respect to societal and individual rights related to pain treatment with regard to safety, efficacy, risks, and benefits. Regulators including the U.S. Food and

Drug Administration (FDA), the Drug Enforcement Agency (DEA), and the Federation of State Medical Boards (FSMB) currently require that when opioid analgesics are considered as part of a pain treatment plan, an analysis not only considers "appropriateness" based on justice toward the individual patient, but also takes into account justice toward other members of the household, members of the community, and other members of society. Undeniably, patients have a justifiable "right" to have their pain and suffering addressed appropriately, but from a societal justice-based perspective, regulators now require that clinicians additionally consider societal-level risks and benefits if opioid analgesics are considered to be an appropriate component of a pain treatment plan.

There have been instances where regulatory decisions have been more heavily weighted toward societal justice, instead of individual justice, with the outcome ultimately impacting available potential clinical treatment options, and to a certain degree, individual justice in terms of access to care. One example is the FDA's decision in 2017 to remove Opana ER® from the market. Opana ER® was an extended-release opioid formulation of oxymorphone with abuse-deterrent properties (i.e., resistant to physical and chemical manipulation), originally approved by the FDA in 2006 and reformulated to an abuse-deterrent formulation by the manufacturer in 2012. The value proposition of an extended-release formulation of an opioid analgesic often is related to a number of factors, including convenience due to less frequent dosing (e.g., twice daily as opposed to four or more times daily), a potentially higher level of adherence due to less frequent dosing, and by virtue of a sustained-release mechanism, potential for a more even level of pain control throughout the course of the day compared to short-acting/immediate-release formulations. However, with these benefits also comes the potential for harm, due to the fact that each unit dose of an extended-release opioid formulation contains more opioid in it, making it more potent, and potentially more dangerous if not taken as directed or if tampered with. This increased potential for harm related to tampering or manipulation of an extended-release formulation led to the development of abuse-deterrent opioid mechanisms to help mitigate the risk of harm resulting from tampering with these more potent medications. These abuse-deterrent formulations were theoretically harder to crush and snort, and more difficult to liquify or inject. This provided clinicians and patients the ability to choose to prescribe these abuse-deterrent opioids when there was increased concern related to the potential for aberrant drug-related behaviors such as tampering, if extended-release opioids were indicated for long-term use. All this was based on justice of the individual needs of the pain patient and consideration of associated risks and benefits of these formulations to the patient.

In a press release in June 2017, the FDA stated that the agency's decision to remove Opana ER from the market was because "the benefits of the drug may no longer outweigh its risks [7]." This statement was referring to a risk/benefit analysis not only for patients, but also for people who might tamper with the pill for purposes such as nonmedical use. The FDA further stated that this was "*the first time the agency has taken steps to remove a currently marketed opioid pain medication from sale due to the public health consequences of abuse. We are facing an opioid epidemic – a public health crisis, and we must take all necessary steps to reduce the scope of opioid misuse and abuse,"* said FDA Commissioner Scott Gottlieb, M.D. *"We will continue to take regulatory steps when we see situations where an opioid product's risks outweigh its benefits, not only for its intended patient population but also in regard to its potential for misuse and abuse."*

The FDA decision was based on postmarketing data which reported that likely because of the abuse-deterrent components of the formulation, nonmedical routes of use of this drug had shifted from snorting it nasally to injecting it intravenously. When used in this fashion, reports of increased incidence of HIV and hepatitis C in substance users began to emerge, likely from an increased incidence of intravenous (IV) use and needle sharing. Additionally, a blood disorder called thrombotic micro-angiopathy (TMA) also began to emerge, related to IV injection of the abuse-deterrent component of the Opana ER, a high-molecular-weight polymer called polyethylene oxide. The complications associated with TMA could be wide ranging, including end-organ damage due to ischemia from occlusion of blood flow. The FDA stated that *"The abuse and manipulation of reformulated Opana ER by injection has resulted in a serious disease outbreak. When we determined that the product had dangerous unintended consequences, we made a decision to request its withdrawal from the market. This action will protect the public from further potential for misuse and abuse of this product."* The FDA also made a commitment to examine all approved opioid analgesics and to take further actions as appropriate with respect to the overdose crisis.

The abovementioned regulatory example is just one where risk to people using an approved pain medication for nonmedical purposes via an unintended route of administration resulted in the removal of the product from the market irrespective of its benefit to patients who used it to control their pain appropriately as directed. In this case, from the perspective of societal justice, risks to people who used the medication nonmedically in an unintended fashion outweighed the individual's right to justice and have access to this particular medication based on patient-level potential risks and benefits. It is a good illustrative example of the intersection and, sometimes potential conflict, that may arise between individual and societal justice.

References

1. Brennan F, Carr DB, Cousins M. Pain management: a fundamental human right. Anesth Analg. 2007;105(1):205–21.
2. Garrett, et al. Health care ethics. 2nd ed. Prentice Hall; 1993.
3. Pain Patient Bill of Rights. The U.S. Pain Foundation. www.uspainfoundation.org. Accessed 10 Feb 2023.
4. Fishman SM. Recognizing pain management as a human right: a first step. Anesth Analg. 2007;105(1):8–9.
5. U.S. Department of Health and Human Services. Pain management best practices inter-agency task force report: updates, gaps, inconsistencies, and recommendations. 2019, May. Retrieved

from U. S. Department of Health and Human Services website: https://www.hhs.gov/ash/advisory-committees/pain/reports/index.html. Accessed 3 July 2023.

6. Snyder JE, Gauthier, CC, Tong R. Evidence-based medical ethics: cases for practice-based learning. Springer Publishing; 2008. ISBN: 978-1-60327-246-9.

7. U.S Food and Drug Administration. FDA requests removal of Opana ER for risks related to abuse. https://www.fda.gov/news-events/press-announcements/fda-requests-removal-opana-er-risks-related-abuse. Accessed 10 July 2023.

Individuality, Choice, and Paternalism in Pain Management

14

Individuality and Pain

For the first time in 41 years, in 2020, the International Association for the Study of Pain (IASP) revised its definition of pain [1]. The motivation for doing so included ensuring that the definition of pain was consistent with progress in scientific evidence and knowledge about pain since its prior definition in 1979, which was accepted globally by clinicians, researchers, professional, governmental, and regulatory agencies including the World Health Organization. Another important goal of the 2020 revised definition was to develop "*a clear, concise, and unambiguous statement that describes the varied experiences of pain, while recognizing its diversity and complexity.*" Additionally, another motivating factor for the IASP to revise the definition of pain was to help clinicians to better understand and recognize pain as a distinct, multifaceted medical condition that is uniquely individual to the person experiencing it, along with helping to improve pain assessment the quality of pain care that people with pain receive.

The updated 2020 IASP definition of pain underscores the idea that **pain is *both* a sensory and emotional experience**, something which was not significantly different from the 1979 definition. But the new definition distinguishes itself significantly in its six qualifying "notes" which reiterate a focus on pain and individuality.

The first note states that "*Pain is always a personal experience, that is influenced to varying degrees by biological, psychological, and social factors.*" This is critical, because it emphasizes the idea that people with the same pathological or physical etiology of pain may have vastly different responses to it from the perspectives of functional impact, quality of life, and level of suffering. Practically, this means that a truly individualized pain assessment and formulation of treatment planning must be informed by these variables to be as tailored to the individual patient as possible.

The second note states that "*Pain and nociception (the central nervous system (CNS) and peripheral nervous system (PNS) processing of painful stimuli) are different phenomena. Pain cannot be inferred solely from activity in sensory*

© The Author(s), under exclusive license to Springer Nature Switzerland AG 2024
K. L. Zacharoff, P. Migdal, *Pain, Drugs, and Ethics*,
https://doi.org/10.1007/978-3-031-63018-7_14

neurons." Clinically, this underscores the need for clinicians to avoid thinking about pain from a purely neurological perspective, or quantified by a simple pain rating (e.g., numerical pain rating scale of 0–10). This particular note may require a significant shift in mindset about pain for both clinicians and patients, and means much more than just the fact that "pain ratings are subjective in nature."

The third note states that "***Through their life experiences, individuals learn the concept of pain***." From the perspective of the pain assessment, there may sometimes be a low level of congruency between pain rating, level of suffering, and functional impact among different patients with pathologically similar painful conditions. This supports the idea that to a certain degree, the way someone thinks about their pain and how they act, process, and experience their pain can be a function of their upbringing, role modeling, and environmental exposure.

The fourth note states that "***A person's report of pain should be respected***." This note refers more to justice, equity, and ethical treatment than individuality, but from a clinical perspective, it means that an individual patient's report of pain, rating of pain, and how pain is impacting their life should be *believed*, respected, and considered to be unique to that person, despite similarities in pathology or other characteristics such as age, physical condition, and overall state of health.

The fifth note states that "***Although pain usually serves an adaptive role, it may have adverse effects on function, social, and psychological well-being***." This note details that some individuals may be more susceptible to developing maladaptive pain, a situation where the protective mechanisms of pain are overridden, and pain becomes "the problem" and less related to associated or actual tissue damage. For example, people who have had poorly treated acute pain may be more likely to develop maladaptive chronic neuropathic pain.

The sixth and final note states that "***Verbal description is only one of several behaviors to express pain; inability to communicate does not negate the possibility that a human or nonhuman animal experiences pain***." People who experience pain may express it differently, and in some cases, not express it at all. It is important to consider *how* patients might report or portray their painful experiences. Additionally, patients who are less or unable to communicate their pain effectively due to age, cognitive impairment, language barriers, or other factors should be equally considered to be experiencing pain as others would be if other evidence suggests this is the case.

A key takeaway from the 2020 revised IASP definition of pain is to recognize that pain is not only a highly subjective experience, but it is also a *highly personal* one as well. In a 2017 article titled "*Individual Differences in Pain: Understanding the Mosaic that Makes Pain Personal*" [2], Fillingim refers to interindividual variability in how people respond to pain due to a "mosaic" of factors that are unique to each individual. Among these factors are **sex differences.** For example, several published studies have demonstrated that chronic pain is more prevalent in women than men [3]. Additionally, research has shown that for all standard measures of experimental pain sensitivity, women display a greater sensitivity to painful stimuli than men, a lower pain threshold, and possibly differences in pain modulation systems. Despite reported differences in magnitude of differences in pain, research shows that the correlation is the same—that women "experience" pain to a greater degree than men. Another factor in the "pain mosaic" is that there can be variability based on **racial/ethnic differences**. Research consistently has shown that both severity and impact of pain is greater in minority patients [4]. While may be difficult to isolate the reasons, the consensus is that there may be a multitude of reasons for these differences, including but not limited socio-economic status and access to pain care [2]. Additionally, minority patients may be at increased risk of undertreatment of pain due to bias and stigma [4], may have differences in pain coping skills, and/or may have genetic differences in pain responses as well [5]. **Age-related differences** in the pain experience can be differentiating factors as well. Unquestionably, with the "aging of America," the number of people 65 and over with pain-related complaints continues to increase and appears to correspond directly with an increased incidence in this patient population of musculoskeletal, neuropathic, and degenerative joint disease. Alternatively, certain types of pain have been shown to decrease in the older patient population as well, such as headache and abdominal pain. It seems that as people age, they may become *less sensitive* to acute painful stimuli, and *more sensitive* to sustained painful stimuli, possibly indicating changes in pain modulation capacity resulting in decreased pain inhibition [6]. Another possible explanation for age-related changes in the pain experience could be the increased incidence of comorbid medical conditions (e.g., diabetes, vascular disease, etc.), reductions in physical activity as one ages, or an increased likelihood of undertreatment due to a number of factors including bias, stigma, or cognitively-impacted communication capacity. It is also important to remember that other possible contributors may include cultural, genetic, hereditary, and psychosocial (e.g., traumatic experiences or developmental influences) differences which can also play a significant role in shaping the personal experience of pain.

From a clinical perspective, this is relevant because it means that a lack of acknowledgement and capture of individual differences in the pain experience could significantly negatively impact pain treatment outcomes. Not considering the intimate relationship between the need to approach the development of a pain treatment plan which incorporates not only biomedical approaches but also biopsychosocial approaches is critical not only in terms of treatment selection, but also in terms of mutually-defined (patient and clinician) realistic goals and expectations of the selected treatment.

Considering individuality in patients with pain could also play a significant role in helping to identify patients who may be more likely to transition from acute to subacute to chronic pain, and to proactively implement tactics and strategies to prevent that transition, not only potentially impacting the patient's future, but also helping to mitigate the significant societal and economic burden of chronic pain as well.

Choice and Pain Management

The delivery of ethical pain care incorporates shared decision-making, which is often defined by the Charles et al. model [7], which identifies core elements of shared decision-making to include that two or more parties are involved in making treatment decisions, that both (or all parties involved) participate in making decisions, that information is shared including available treatment options and their individual risks and benefits (i.e., informed consent), and that there is congruency among the decision-makers about the ultimate treatment plan implementation.

As discussed many times throughout this text, mutually-determined (clinician-patient/caregiver) pain treatment planning has the most likely chance of producing favorable pain treatment outcomes, higher levels of adherence, patient satisfaction, increased efficacy, clinician gratification, and likely, safety. Unfortunately, many things today have the potential to become barriers to patient's, clinician's, and caregiver's ability to make autonomous decisions about pain treatment. There is likely no greater illustration of a potential barrier than the use of, or appropriateness of, opioid analgesic therapy and insurance coverage of possible alternative nonopioid pain treatment options. With a majority of people with pain managed in a primary care setting, this can present a multitude of challenges for those clinicians and their patients in a number of different ways. Often, a lack of foundational education about pain and its management places nonexpert frontline practitioners at a significant disadvantage, with their clinical approaches dictated by healthcare system-level pain treatment algorithms, fear of regulatory scrutiny about opioid prescribing at the regional level, federal level, or both, and in many cases the omnipresent challenge of managing efficiency in pain care delivery. Shared decision-making about pain treatment options can be time-consuming, and requires not only an awareness of constraints and communication about them, but also mutual understanding.

Pain is one of *the* most common reasons that adults in the United States seek medical attention [8]. It therefore might seem logical that 24 years after designating pain as the 5th vital sign in 2000, there would be a greater level of durable consensus with respect to pain treatment instead of seemingly never-ending debates about how patients should best be managed as safely and effectively as possible, based on evidence, science, clinical observations, and patient-based case reports. Instead, in many cases, the scientific evidence basis is lacking, and a desired level of congruency does not often exist with respect to pain treatment and the facilitation of informed and consistent shared decision-making.

There have been numerous waves of recommendations for the "*best*" options to treat people with pain, many with respect to the treatment of chronic pain, but also are appropriate for the treatment of most types of pain. The 2019 Department of Health and Human Services *Pain Management Best Practices Inter-Agency Task Force Report: Updates, Gaps, Inconsistencies, and Recommendations (HHS Report)* [9] distills pain treatment recommendations down to **five major types of treatment options** that should ethically be considered options as components of a pain treatment plan when appropriate and identified and selected through shared decision-making.

The first category of treatment options recommended in the HHS Report involves the use of **pharmacotherapeutic agents** (often the most commonly utilized pain treatment option by a large margin), which can be categorized into two broad categories; **nonopioid** (e.g., acetaminophen, nonsteroidal anti-inflammatory drugs, anticonvulsants, musculoskeletal agents, anxiolytics) and **opioid** analgesic medications. Each medication in either category has its own inherent risk-benefit profile, mechanism of action, inclusive of the patient's individual risk benefit profile determined by their medical history, biopsychosocial history, and life context including goals and expectations, duties, and activities of daily living. In many cases, multimodal pharmacologic therapy, incorporating one or more medications can be employed for a number of reasons including a desire to capitalize on synergistic effects (e.g., anti-inflammatory, and pain-relieving), or an effort to decrease the amount of opioid prescribed and possible opioid-related adverse effects (opioid-sparing).

The second category of treatment options mentioned in this HHS Report involves the use of **restorative therapies**, which typically include physical treatments that are often complementary to pharmacotherapy, such as physical or occupational therapy, exercise programs, transcutaneous electric nerve stimulation (TENS), massage therapy, thermal treatments, ultrasonic therapy, and traction or bracing. The value proposition for these types of therapy is paramount in two ways: one being that they are often rooted in the goal of maintaining and/or improving functionality in the face of pain, and the other being that they often involve patient motivation and participation. A major hindrance, and something that needs to be realistically considered in the shared decision-making process with the patient, is the question of insurance coverage and reimbursement. The report recommends that policymakers *"closely evaluate and advocate for payers to improve access to a range of restorative therapies."* Recommending a restorative therapeutic treatment may not be a viable option if the patient is not able to afford it, it is not likely to be covered by their insurance, or both.

The third category of pain treatment options in the HHS Report involves the use of **interventional procedures**, encompassing minimally invasive procedures that can sometimes be used to treat pain effectively, and help to complement, or in some cases eliminate, the need for pharmacotherapy. Often, the more complex procedures are typically performed by expert-level clinicians, and their availability or patient volume can possibly be an issue from a realistic and logistical perspective. In some cases, interventional procedures are not only used therapeutically, but also may be used for diagnostic purposes, helping to hone in on the pathophysiologic or mechanistic causes of pain. Epidural steroid injections are one example of interventional pain procedures and have been used for many years to help to treat many different types of back pain. Over the years there have been "pendulum swings" (for or against) with respect to their efficacy [10] and safety [11], but many clinicians, patients, and clinical reports [12] attest to their utility as part of the pain management armamentarium for treating certain types of back pain. Other interventional pain management procedures include trigger point injections, intraarticular injections, peripheral nerve injections, neuro-ablations, and spinal cord stimulation. Similar to restorative therapies, reimbursement and insurance should be an important issue to consider with respect to interventional procedures as a potential choice for pain treatment.

The fourth category of pain treatment options in the HHS Report is comprised of **behavioral health approaches**, which take into consideration the intimate relationship between the biomedical and biopsychosocial aspects of the pain experience. These approaches are numerous and include cognitive behavioral therapy, behavioral therapy, acceptance and commitment therapy, mindfulness and stress reduction, and biofeedback to name a few. Like other components of a multidisciplinary approach to pain treatment, access to these interventions, insurance coverage, and reimbursement for them can sometimes be major barriers to their use as a viable pain treatment choice. The 2019 HHS Report recommends that utilizing these approaches in novel ways could counter some of these barriers, such as using telehealth as a mode of delivery, mobile apps to facilitate self-directed programs, public awareness campaigns to educate the public about the efficacy of these approaches, and improvements with respect to payer coverage and reimbursement. Additionally, the report stresses the importance of healthcare professional education about the value proposition of these modalities to help future clinicians have an understanding of the biopsychosocial aspects of pain and the important role of behavioral health approaches as complementary components of a pain treatment plan.

The fifth category of pain treatment options in the HHS Report consists of a variety of **complementary and integrative health approaches**. Complementary approaches are commonly just that—complements to "traditional" treatments such as pharmacotherapy and physical treatments and are meant to be used in conjunction to those treatments as opposed to alternatives to them. These include mind-body interventions, acupuncture, massage therapy, osteopathic and chiropractic manipulation, meditation/movement therapies (e.g., yoga), and naturopathic products and dietary supplements. Integrative health approaches involve the coordination of common and complementary pain treatments in a coordinated fashion. In some cases, there is a substantial amount about of scientific evidence about the safety and efficacy of these treatments, and in other cases it may be lacking, but in light of the overdose crisis, there is an increased desire to have clinicians and patients rely less heavily on pharmacotherapy, particularly opioid analgesics as much as possible [13]. Once again, these strategies rely heavily on the education of clinicians, health system administrators, and the public with respect to the utility of these approaches, and about the need for advocacy for their insurance coverage and reimbursement by payers as well.

According to the 2019 HHS Report, all the abovementioned categories of pain treatment approaches are informed and affected by four critical topics, which are always important to consider. Regardless of the approach(es) considered, **a detailed risk assessment** which provides the clinician and patient with the potential risks and benefits is essential. This analysis needs to be individualized and directed toward function, quality of life, ability to perform activities of daily living, and realistic expectations of adherence, requiring mutual deliberation and communication. **Stigma** is another critically important concern. It is not uncommon for people with chronic pain to feel stigmatized, and even more common if their pain is being treated with a pharmacotherapeutic approach that includes opioid analgesics [14, 15]. The consequences of stigma and discrimination are real, and can be substantial, and potentially disabling; they may include feelings of guilt, shame, judgment, and embarrassment which may lead many negative outcomes including anxiety, depression, loss of self-worth, social isolation, and a lower likelihood of adherence to the pain treatment plan. **Access to care** affects the likelihood of success of any pain treatment option, and it is equally important to consider disparate patient populations in this equation. These populations include but are not limited to children, older adults, cognitively impaired individuals, women, patients with comorbid chronic pain conditions such as cancer or sickle cell disease, members of racial and ethnic minorities, and people involved in active service in the military or veterans. Lastly, and repeatedly underscored throughout the HHS Report is the dictum that **education is one of the most significant factors that impact pain and its treatment.** Educational deficits about pain management, risk assessment, stigma, discrimination, opioid analgesics, substance use disorder, and virtually every related topic have the potential to negatively impact pain treatment at virtually every level, including the general public, clinicians, patients, healthcare system administrators, policymakers, legislators, regulators, and law enforcement officials. The HHS recommends a "**sea change**" in academic centers, health systems, regulatory agencies (Federal, State, and Local), and insurers with respect to educating *all* stakeholders with the intention of achieving an improved ethical balance to the delivery of pain care, along with maximizing safety and efficacy of pain treatments.

The intersection of the overdose epidemic and the utility of opioid analgesics has had significant impact on mutually derived (clinician and patient) pain treatment planning; in many cases because of regulatory efforts to reduce the soaring number of drug-related overdose deaths each year (more than 107,000 in 2021) [16]. With over 1,000,000 people losing their lives to drug overdoses in the past 24 years [17], the term "crisis" unquestionably applies. And it is important to point out that approximately 66% of these overdose deaths involved an opioid, and that when surveyed, an overwhelming majority of substance users reported that their first substance of unhealthy use was a prescription pain medication (i.e., opioid analgesic). However, it is also important to note that in most cases, the substance user was *__not__* the person to whom the opioids were prescribed. Often the drugs were obtained from a family member, a friend, or access to a family member or friend's prescribed medication which was not stored in a secure and safe location (e.g., medicine cabinet) or an illicit channel of distribution, such as a drug dealer.

The question then becomes whether or not the people succumbing to overdose fatalities are most likely patients to whom opioids were prescribed to treat their pain or not, and whether regulatory decisions made to limit options available for clinician and patient shared decision-making are ethical. Certainly, regulatory decisions have been made on that point. At least since the release of the 2016 CDC Guidelines for opioid prescribing (mentioned many times throughout this book), the regulatory charge has been to decrease the number of opioid prescriptions written and/or amount dispensed. Passionate arguments have been made at public regulatory meetings (e.g., U.S. Food and Drug Administration Advisory Committee Meetings) and on social media on both sides of these regulatory efforts. Many people (clinical experts and laypeople) have argued that opioids are not likely necessary in the majority of patients for whom they are prescribed, that they are much more addictive than initially thought, and that many people would still be alive today if it were not for opioid analgesics. Alternatively, via these same platforms, many patients with chronic pain have argued that if opioid analgesics were not available to them, their level of function, quality of life, and pain ratings would be substantially worse and ultimately life-limiting. Additionally, patients often report the end-result of limiting opioid prescribing and availability, where in some cases, clinicians tell them that their opioids must be forcibly tapered, discontinued, or simply that they must seek out someone else to get their opioids prescribed. Since the release of the 2016 CDC Opioid Guidelines [18], the idea of an opioid "ceiling dose" has been another heated ethical issue of contention and debate; potentially limiting choices for some patients being treated with opioid analgesics. Despite the recommendation in the 2016 guidelines that in nonexpert clinical settings the daily dose limit should not exceed 90 morphine milligram equivalents (MME), there is not a substantiated scientific foundation for that limitation recommendation, and it does not take into account the fact that the therapeutic window needs to be individualized for every patient and can vary significantly. A study by Dasgupta et al. [19] evaluated the risk of mortality related to opioid dose in over 2 million patients in North Carolina and found that the mortality rate was low. These researchers reported that: "*Dose-dependent opioid overdose risk among patients increased gradually and did not show evidence of a distinct risk threshold. Much of the risk at higher doses appears to be associated with co-prescribed benzodiazepines. It is critical to account for overlapping prescriptions and justifies taking a person-time approach to MME calculation with intent-to-treat principles.*"

The purpose of making these points is that while it does seem as if there are numerous choices available to clinicians and patients to mutually determine the best course of action when constructing a pain treatment plan, in reality there are **a number of constraints** which potentially limit the realistic choices actually available. **Access to expert-level care** may be unrealistic due to geographic variables such as distance and availability of expert-level clinical resources. While telemedicine has made progress in that regard with respect to consultation and assessment, it has not solved the issue of offering interventional treatment options when logistical challenges exist. The 2019 HHS Report consistently identifies the fact that complex pain management situations (e.g., more than just pharmacotherapy) are often hindered by challenges related to **insurance coverage and reimbursement**. These challenges include lack of insurance, insufficient coverage, and most importantly issues related to reimbursement for non-pharmacologic pain treatment approaches such as behavioral and other complementary options mentioned above. Inherent in the reimbursement system is a lack of guidance from insurers with respect to data needed to determine qualification for coverage and reimbursement of non-medical pain treatments. The HHS Report states that "*The inconsistencies in insurance policies, the variability in guidance regarding coverage determinations, and the variability in utilization management tools that coverage providers use can cause delays in service delivery, provision of inadequate treatment, and added financial and* *psychosocial burden for patients with pain.*" This also may ultimately choose less attractive and less optimal treatment choices.

In the final analysis, for the multitude of multimodal and multidisciplinary pain treatment options that exist, it often seems as if the choices for pain treatment in the real world may actually be quite limited for many clinicians and their patients. It is not uncommon that the most "cost effective" choice for pain treatment is/are the one(s) that is/are biomedical and pharmacologic, and not biopsychosocial and complementary in nature. In fact, ironically, despite everything mentioned about the intersection of the overdose epidemic and the use (or overuse) of opioid analgesics to treat pain, opioids may often be the default choice, because in many cases they are often the least expensive choice, which is something that payers find attractive. Alternatively, as mentioned many times throughout the course of this book, regulatory efforts may further limit the available choices because of the desire to limit opioid prescribing as a strategy for decreasing overdose fatalities. Things can become a bit "sketchy" with respect to the use of opioid analgesics to treat pain. Typically, in the practice of medicine, it is recommended that for any patient-centered treatment planning, there should always be a good "Plan B" included as part of that plan in case an alternative is needed or desired. Pain management is no different than other areas of medicine in that regard; however, it is not uncommon today to have "Plan A" be to avoid opioids, with "Plan B" being either unclear or undefined altogether—in many cases the end-result is *the opposite of choice*. Additionally, patients may often be confused about the unwillingness of some clinicians to utilize opioids, and in most cases, unaware of regulatory efforts to curb prescribing them. Communication could go a long way to helping to refocus shared decision-making to make sure that patients understand the forces at play outside of the clinical encounter which may limit available potential pain treatment options. This communication should not only include issues about opioid prescribing, but also requires attention to what other potential treatments might or might not be reimbursed, covered at all, or available to patients with no insurance at all.

Paternalism in Pain Management

Most clinical training programs teach their students that paternalism in medicine is an outdated, unethical, and unprofessional approach to health care which has little or no place in the practice of modern medicine. **Clinical paternalism** is commonly defined as the clinician making decisions about a course or courses of treatment in the absence of informed consent, without understanding and shared decision-making. As mentioned previously in another chapter, future clinicians are taught today that autonomy is the favored approach, and that whenever possible patient involvement in decision-making (shared decision-making) is key to the delivery of ethical care [20]. This rationale is well supported in scientific literature demonstrating the positive effects of autonomy and shared decision-making including improved treatment outcomes, a higher level of adherence to treatment regimens, better coping skills, and patient satisfaction [21]. A more in-depth analysis of the benefits of patient autonomy reveals a higher sense of respect between clinician and patient, along with a higher level of investment and motivation.

In the context of pain management, it is important to consider that it is not uncommon for patients in pain to present with the request to the clinician to "*just get rid of my pain*" or "*just make my pain go away.*" Further affirming a desire for paternalistic treatment with the patient stating, "*I'll do whatever you say if you can make this pain better, just tell me what to do.*" It is also not uncommon for clinicians to advise patients to "*just do what I say, and your pain will get better.*" As illustrated earlier in this chapter, treatment planning for pain management has become quite complex, and with so many different forces at play impacting the possible courses of treatment, it might not be realistically possible to achieve the highest level of autonomy and shared decision-making completely devoid of any paternalistic influence on pain treatment planning altogether. Additionally, very often pain is accompanied by suffering, and for people who are actively suffering, active participation in shared decision-making may be impractical to expect due to distress and sometimes may be the last thing that patients are interested in beyond pain relief. Sometimes what patients in pain may be looking for from their clinician is just the right balance between autonomy, beneficence, nonmaleficence, justice, and some "**selective paternalism**" [21] for choosing the "best" components of a pain treatment plan. Selective paternalism is defined as the strategic use of paternalism when autonomous and shared decision-making is not realistically practical.

In 1992, Ezekiel and Linda Emanuel identified **four models of the physician-patient relationship** which represent different perspectives about paternalism and its potential role in the ethical delivery of medical care and are relevant today with respect to how there could be blending of paternalism in the ethical delivery of pain care [22]. The first model is the **paternalistic model**, where as described above, the clinician uses objective information to make determinations about the best course of action based on their opinion of what is "best for the patient." Next is the **scientific or informative model**, based on more of a "consumer" model of healthcare. The clinician's job is to provide the facts to the patient without imposing their values into the decision-making process but providing expertise in helping the patient make a completely autonomous decision about the desired course(s) of action. Another model is the **interpretive model**, which is based on the desire of the clinician to determine the patient's values and goals with the intention of helping the patient select the possible treatment options to achieve those goals taking into account risks and benefits of those options. This model rests upon the ability of the clinician to capture an adequate patient narrative that facilitates the identification of those values and goals as they may sometimes be unknown to the patient. Lastly is the **deliberative model**, which involves the clinician helping the patient choose the best health-related values that can possibly be achieved based on the individual patient circumstances, helping the patient identify what the best course(s) of action would be based on the clinician's opinion of what is best based on communication and discussion of worthiness of possible treatment options based solely on the worthiness of those options based on health-related values, and not moral or judgmental ones.

It may very well be that one of the Emanuel's models may be more appropriate for certain patients than others, and it may also be true that some blend of all four of these models mentioned may be the most appropriate and ethical approach based on the individual patient, their values, their goals, and the likelihood of achieving the best pain treatment outcomes possible. What is important is to consider *all* these as possibilities.

References

1. Raja SN, Carr DB, Cohen M, Finnerup NB, Flor H, Gibson S, Keefe FJ, Mogil JS, Ringkamp M, Sluka KA, Song XJ, Stevens B, Sullivan MD, Tutelman PR, Ushida T, Vader K. The revised International Association for the Study of Pain definition of pain: concepts, challenges, and compromises. Pain. 2020;161(9):1976–82.
2. Fillingim RB. Individual differences in pain: understanding the mosaic that makes pain personal. Pain. 2017;158(Suppl 1):S11–8.
3. Fillingim RB, King CD, Ribeiro-Dasilva MC, Rahim-Williams B, Riley JL 3rd. Sex, gender, and pain: a review of recent clinical and experimental findings. J Pain. 2009 May;10(5):447–85.
4. Morales ME, Yong RJ. Racial and ethnic disparities in the treatment of chronic pain. Pain Med. 2021;22(1):75–90.
5. Rahim-Williams B, Riley JL 3rd, Williams AK, Fillingim RB. A quantitative review of ethnic group differences in experimental pain response: do biology, psychology, and culture matter? Pain Med. 2012;13(4):522–40.
6. Fillingim RB. Individual differences in pain responses. Curr Rheumatol Rep. 2005;7(5):342–7.
7. Ref-Charles C, Gafni A, Whelan T. Shared decision-making in the medical encounter: what does it mean? (or it takes at least two to tango). Soc Sci Med. 1997;44(5):681–92.
8. Yong RJ, Mullins PM, Bhattacharyya N. Prevalence of chronic pain among adults in the United States. Pain. 2022;163(2):e328–32.
9. U.S. Department of Health and Human Services. Pain management best practices interagency task force report: updates, gaps, inconsistencies, and recommendations. (2019, May). Retrieved from U. S. Department of Health and Human Services website: https://www.hhs.gov/ash/advisory-committees/pain/reports/index.html. Accessed 3 July 2023.
10. Shelton S, Yochum ADO, Walker E, Waters N. Effectiveness of epidural steroid injections for low Back pain. Am Fam Physician. 2022 Jul;106(1):89–90.
11. Bicket MC, Chakravarthy K, Chang D, Cohen SP. Epidural steroid injections: an updated review on recent trends in safety and complications. Pain Manag. 2015;5(2):129–46.
12. Pandey RA. Efficacy of epidural steroid injection in management of lumbar prolapsed intervertebral disc: a comparison of caudal, transforaminal and interlaminar routes. J Clin Diagn Res. 2016;10(7):RC05-11.
13. Tick H, Nielsen A, Pelletier KR, Bonakdar R, Simmons S, Glick R, Ratner E, Lemmon RL, Wayne P, Zador V; Pain task force of the academic consortium for integrative medicine and health. Evidence-based nonpharmacologic strategies for comprehensive pain care: the consortium pain task force White paper. Explore (NY). 2018;14(3):177–211.
14. McAllister MJ. How to end the stigma of pain. https://instituteforchronicpain.org/understanding-chronic-pain/healthcare-system-failings/how-to-end-the-stigma-of-pain. Accessed 14 July 2023.
15. Slade SC, Molloy E, Keating JL. Stigma experienced by people with nonspecific chronic low back pain: a qualitative study. Pain Med. 2009;10(1):143–54.
16. Centers for Disease Control and Prevention. Drug overdose deaths remain high. https://www.cdc.gov/drugoverdose/deaths/index.html#print. Accessed 14 July 2023.
17. Spencer MR, Miniño AM, Warner M. Drug overdose deaths in the United States, 2001–2021, NCHS Data Brief, no 457. Hyattsville: National Center for Health Statistics. p. 2022.

18. Dowell D, Haegerich TM, Chou R. CDC guideline for prescribing opioids for chronic pain — United States, 2016. MMWR Recomm Rep. 2016;65(RR-1):1–49.
19. Dasgupta N, Funk MJ, Proescholdbell S, Hirsch A, Ribisl KM, Marshall S. Cohort study of the impact of high-dose opioid analgesics on overdose mortality. Pain Med. 2016;17(1):85–98.
20. Bailoor K, Valley T, Perumalswami C, Shuman AG, DeVries R, Zahuranec DB. How acceptable is paternalism? A survey-based study of clinician and nonclinician opinions on paternalistic decision making. AJOB Empir Bioeth. 2018;9(2):91–8.
21. Drolet BC, White CL. Selective paternalism. Virtual Mentor. 2012;14(7):582–8.
22. Emanuel EJ, Emanuel LL. Four models of the physician-patient relationship. JAMA. 1992;267(16):2221–6.

Ethics, Opioids, and the Overdose Epidemic

15

Ethics and Opioids

There has been so much "motion" or flux with respect to the use of opioid analgesics to treat pain since 2000, that the phrase "**The Opioid Pendulum**" was coined to label it. This term refers to the change from a time "liberal" prescribing of opioids (**opiophilia**) to a period with more discriminating, restrictive, or "conservative" prescribing of opioids (**opiophobia**). A visit to the National Capital Poison Center (Poison Control) website [1] defines the opioid pendulum as *"the oscillation between over-prescribing and under-prescribing of opioids."* The reason this definition resonates with me is because it implies that neither side of the swinging pendulum has been "good" from an ethical perspective, but more like a "Goldilocks fashion," too much one way, or too much the other way, with neither being "just right."

As we begin to look at what has happened over the past 24+ years in the United States, it is important to consider that in the late 1990s, it was not uncommon for clinicians (most commonly physicians at that time) to be successfully litigated against for malpractice for not treating or under-treating someone's pain. I was there, and it was happening. In some cases, these lawsuits were brought forward by caregivers or family members of elderly or infirm people who felt that their loved ones suffered due to their pain unnecessarily. At that time (and still today), most clinicians tasked with caring for people with pain were frontline, nonexpert (i.e., *not* pain specialists), primary care practitioners, such as Family Medicine Physicians, Internal Medicine Specialists, etc.

In 2000, when pain was designated the 5th vital sign, the pain rating (e.g., Numerical Rating Scale (NRS) 0-10) was elevated to a status on par with pulse, respiratory rate, blood pressure, and temperature. I remember thinking about the challenge(s) this could present to clinicians who had received little to no education about the pathophysiology of pain, how to uniformly perform a comprehensive pain assessment, and how to develop a pain treatment plan, especially one that incorporated the use of opioid analgesics. Basically, I watched the numerical pain scale

© The Author(s), under exclusive license to Springer Nature Switzerland AG 2024
K. L. Zacharoff, P. Migdal, *Pain, Drugs, and Ethics*,
https://doi.org/10.1007/978-3-031-63018-7_15

(NRS) 0–10, with 0 being no pain at all, and 10 being pain as bad as it could be, become **the thing** to treat—the goal being to lower that number. Once clinicians were given a mandate to ask virtually all patients about their pain, it would need to be documented, and something would need to be reflected in the medical record with respect to what was being done to address it. "Clinical paternalism" was more prevalent at that time than it is today, and often the goals and metrics of successful pain treatment in clinician's minds were not necessarily in alignment with those of the patient. It is not hard to imagine that patients wanted their pain rating to be reduced to 0, and clinicians just wanted to see it *improvement*, with no good foundational training or evidence basis about what degree of decrease should be considered significant improvement. Some articles and guidelines in the literature stated that if the pain rating could be lowered by 33%, it would be a satisfactory level of progress. Other guidances stated that the goal should be any pain rating ≤ 5 (based on an NRS 0–10), while others stated that a 2–3-point reduction in patient pain ratings was a "win." At the time, there was no significant mention of function, and little or no mention of quality of life or the ability to perform activities of daily living, which could have at least led to individualized goals and expectations of "success" to some degree. The goal in those days was to treat "the number," which obviously was completely subjective and, in some ways, essentially meaningless. There were patients who rated their pain at a 4, and could not get up off the sofa to get to the clinic, work, or perform activities of daily living, and others who reported that their pain was a 9 or 10, and that they could not get the clinic until after they were done with a day's work.

So *how* did clinicians respond to this elevation of pain to vital sign status and the need to treat the pain rating? In many cases, *with their prescription pads.* In many cases, when people sought medical attention to address their pain, they had more than likely already self-treated with over-the-counter medications that they had at home—they came expecting that prescription for "something stronger." And when prescriptions were indeed written, they were often not prescription-strength versions of medications that patients likely had already taken to self-treat their pain (e.g., nonsteroidal anti-inflammatory drugs (NSAIDs), acetaminophen), these prescriptions were commonly for opioid analgesics. Prescribers knew that opioids could treat pain and suffering for a multitude of pain types, and patients considered that leaving the office with a prescription pain medication was the "reward" for taking the time and effort to seek medical attention for their pain and ease their suffering. There was also no framework for what quantity of opioid should be supplied in the prescription, just the idea that what nobody wanted was for the patient to run out of it on a weekend evening, prompting a call to the prescriber to prescribe more, so more than an ample amount would often be supplied. We will get to the impact of this point a bit later in this chapter. Suffice it to say that once pain was designated the 5th vital sign, opioids were being prescribed in response to the seemingly ever-increasing number of patients who had pain-related complaints.

Ethics, Opioids, and Blame

As mentioned previously in this book, there has been a lot of conjecture and "finger-pointing" with respect to *who* promoted the elevation of pain to "vital sign status." Some say most of the blame rests on the shoulders of manufacturers of opioids, and that the elevation of pain to vital sign status was a slick marketing strategy to encourage more prescriptions for their medications (e.g., opioid analgesics) to be written, with the intention of increasing revenues. It certainly would be difficult to say that manufacturers of opioids are free from blame in terms of what followed the designation of pain as a vital sign. Indisputably, *pharmaceutical companies have played a significant role in the story of increased opioid prescribing since 2000*, with some manufacturers having been found in violation of a multitude of regulatory restrictions, including but not limited to promoting messaging which downplayed the addictive nature of opioid analgesics, and in certain situations marketing them to prescribers for off-label uses (uses that deviate from the product labeling, which is prohibited by the Food and Drug Administration, FDA). It is also worth noting that for at least the first decade of the 2000s, most if not all education available to clinicians in practice about managing pain was developed, delivered, and funded by these very same pharmaceutical manufacturers, a phenomenon which in many cases still exists today. This education was largely "nonpromotional," which means that it did not contain marketing materials or promotional messaging and was "certified" as being free of conflict and to meet the criteria continuing medical education programming. This education was often presented by many of *the most respected pain experts* at the time, which afforded it a significant level of credibility. For clinicians who had little to no education on the subject and who were shouldering most patients seeking medical attention for their pain, it was often very impactful for them at the time to be exposed to respected, widely known pain experts, and their perspectives and recommendations. Currently, there has been a significant shift in perspective retrospectively regarding the experts' participation in those educational programs, citing that even though the material presented was indeed "nonpromotional" in nature and accredited to provide continuing education, it actually was in many cases, a type of marketing. There are many who retrospectively feel that these experts, who were often very well compensated for their participation in these educational programs, while lending credibility to the education, were delivering messaging that was crafted by the manufacturers to subliminally promote increased opioid prescribing. In fact, when several states across the United States filed lawsuits against opioid manufacturers for their role in creating the "opioid epidemic," some of the more well-known expert lecturers who delivered the education were named as co-defendants in these lawsuits as well. It is beyond the scope of this chapter, but a quick Internet search will detail the flurry of lawsuits and settlements against pharmaceutical companies, pharmaceutical distributors, pharmacy chains, and pain experts who were frequent participants in these industry-created educational programs.

A number of researchers, patient advocacy groups, and healthcare and healthcare-related systems readily embraced the designation of pain as the 5th vital sign as well. Many blame (or give credit to, depending on their viewpoint) the **American Pain Society (APS)** as *the* organization responsible for initiating the idea that pain should be considered as "the 5th vital sign." Many different speeches, writings, and presentations given by prominent members of these pain advocacy groups and research organizations are referred to as laying the groundwork for the idea of designating pain rating as a "vital sign." Virtually every pain advocacy organization aligned themselves with this idea at the time, along with promoting safe and effective use of opioid analgesics to treat pain. In fact, in 2009, **the American Pain Society and the American Academy of Pain Medicine (AAPM)** developed a joint set of guidelines for the use of opioid analgesics for the treatment of chronic non-cancer pain [2]. These guidelines were developed by these respected organizations with the intention of promoting safe and effective use of opioids to treat pain and were created by some of the most respected clinicians and researchers in the field of pain management. The APS/AAPM guidelines stressed the notion that opioids *could* be potentially valuable in certain patients with chronic pain, but also *carried significant risks* related to adverse effects and a high potential for nonmedical use aberrant drug-related behaviors, and addiction. These guidelines were the product of a careful review of the literature for evidence basis, and stressed the importance of identifying patients at increased risk, the importance of informed consent as part of the opioid prescribing process, how patients should be carefully monitored while on opioid therapy, and also detailed contingencies for exit strategies in the event that discontinuation of opioid therapy was indicated. Unfortunately, these guidelines were not widely disseminated to the nonexpert clinicians who could have potentially benefited from this kind of guidance—frontline practitioners. Once again, when litigation brought by many states against pharmaceutical manufacturers, distributors, etc., the American Pain Society was often also named as a co-defendant, in many cases, because of the fact that the APS had received significant amounts of industry sponsorship over the course of its existence from opioid manufacturers. The lawsuits mentioned numerous concerns about messaging which could have been interpreted to have been promoting the use of opioids and contributing to the overdose crisis that ensued. In fact, some referred to the APS as a "pawn of big pharma" that helped to promote pain as the 5th vital sign, which then led to overprescribing of opioids. In addition to the litigation, a report from the U.S. Senate Homeland Security and Governmental Affairs Committee [3] stated that "*Many of the groups discussed in this report have amplified or issued messages that reinforce industry efforts to promote opioid prescription and use, including guidelines and policies minimizing the risk of addiction and promoting opioids for chronic pain.*" This report specifically stated that the abovementioned 2009 joint guidelines issued by American Pain Society and the American Academy of Pain Medicine "promoted opioids as 'safe and effective'," concluding "*…that organizations receiving substantial funding from manufacturers have, in fact, amplified and reinforced messages favoring increased opioid use. By aligning medical culture with industry goals in this way, many of the groups described above may have played a significant role in creating the necessary conditions for the U.S. opioid epidemic.*" Despite its well-respected reputation for education and promotion of research to better treat people with pain safely and effectively, the APS filed for bankruptcy in 2019 and ceased operations due to inability to sustain the legal costs associated with its defense in the thousands of lawsuits which included it as a co-defendant.

The **American Pain Foundation (APF)**, a well-known and highly regarded pain patient advocacy organization ceased operations in 2012 as well for similar reasons to those that led to the demise of the APS, with investigations yielding estimates that as much as 90% of its revenue came from industry sponsors (e.g., drug and/or device manufacturers) amid accusations that the organization was actually "a shill" for promoting opioid manufacturer messaging and increased prescribing. It is important to note that it was not uncommon for drug manufacturers to provide economic support to patient advocacy organizations related to their respective "disease space," and this continues to be the case today. But the development of the overdose epidemic yielded pressure on the APF which was too great, and because they did not have the funds to defend themselves in the numerous lawsuits in which they were named, resulted in a fate similar to that of the APS.

The **American Cancer Society (ACS)** also played a pivotal role in pain being designated the 5th vital sign, because at the time there was a recognition of a significant need for advocacy for patients with cancer-related pain, which was highly prevalent in patients with cancer. Many other patient advocacy groups joined with ACS in advocating for all patients to have the right to have their pain appropriately assessed and treated. **The Veterans Health Administration** is often cited as embracing pain as the 5th vital sign as evidenced in its October 2000 *Pain as the Fifth Vital Sign Toolkit* [4], stating that "*the toolkit has been designed to promote Pain as the 5th Vital Sign and to offer guidelines for the completion of comprehensive pain assessments. These are the initial steps in promoting and improving pain management for veterans receiving care within the VHA system.*" The toolkit went on to state that "*It is important to emphasize that 'Pain as the 5th Vital Sign' is a screening mechanism for identifying unrelieved pain. Screening for pain can be administered quickly for most patients on a routine basis. As with any other vital sign, a positive pain score should trigger further assessment of the pain, prompt intervention, and follow-up evaluation of the pain and the effectiveness of treatment.*"

The Joint Commission (JC), a nonprofit organization which accredits more than 22,000 health care organizations and clinical settings (mainly hospitals) is not free from blame by many either. In 2000, the JC published standards for pain management [5] underscoring the need to improve care related to the "invisible" condition of pain. These standards included conducting quantitative assessments of pain (pain rating on a numerical rating scale, e.g., 0–10). At the time, these standards were lauded by pain experts as a step in the right direction to improve pain care. According to the JC, the reaction was an overreliance on the numerical pain assessment, and that the consensus was that "*Pain became the enemy that needed to be eradicated.*" There were also concerns that JC inspections of clinic settings could be negative, unless policies and procedures were shown to be in place which met the JC's benchmarks for pain treatment. The JC began to revise its standards and removed the requirement for pain assessment from its standards in 2009, in 2011 adding to its recommendations that pain should be treated with both pharmacologic and nonpharmacologic modalities, and in 2016 drafted completely new wording (approved in 2017) which added that caution needed to be taken to ensure "*safe and* *judicious prescribing of opioids*." But many feel that by then, the damage had been done. Patients had been given "the right" to be satisfied with respect to the treatment of their pain, and opioids were the "go to" treatment.

The Federation of State Medical Boards (FSMB) and the Drug Enforcement Administration (DEA) also issued statements to address blame fear among clinicians related to concerns of regulatory scrutiny for prescribing opioids for the sake of treating pain, the 5th vital sign [6].

A report from the Offices of Congressional Representatives Katherine Clark and Hal Rogers was published in 2019 [7], titled *Corrupting the Influence: Purdue the WHO*. As the title implies, this report details concerns among members of Congress that the **World Health Organization (WHO)** was being influenced by the manufacturer of Oxycontin® to "*expand their drug sales to international marketing using the same fraudulent marketing tactics that instigated the opioid crisis in the United States.*" Although the 5th vital sign was not directly mentioned in this report, it focused on the messaging from the WHO, which endorsed the use of opioids to treat both adults with noncancer-related pain and children with persistent pain with opioid analgesics to be essentially "marketing materials for Purdue Pharmaceuticals."

As stated earlier in this chapter, there was so much happening with respect to the call to better treat patients with pain, and pain being designated the 5th vital sign, that clinicians responded by prescribing pain medications—*opioid pain medications*. But something else was happening as well. Nefarious clinicians were capitalizing on pain becoming the 5th vital sign, and the call for better pain treatment by selling prescription opioid medications for profit; they were operating **"pill mills."** The "leader of the pack" in terms of pill mills at the time was the state of **Florida**. A 2019 *Associated Press* article by Terry Spencer was appropriately titled *Florida "Pill Mills" were the "Gas on the Fire" of Opioid Crisis* [8]. This article detailed how and why Florida held the leading title, identifying that in 2010, 90 of the country's top 100 opioid prescribers were in the state of Florida. Additionally, other reports stated that more opioid prescriptions were written in Florida than in the other 49 states in the United States combined. It was not uncommon for people from all over the country to travel to Florida just to obtain opioid prescriptions which could be sold illicitly, many of these people from Ohio, Kentucky, and West Virginia. In fact, and award-winning 2009 documentary about this phenomenon titled *The Oxycontin Express* referred to people routinely traveling to Florida for the sole purpose of obtaining opioids which could then be used for nonmedical purposes or sold on the street for a significant profit to substance users. Many factors contributed to the proliferation of these pill mills, including the fact that it was legal at the time for prescribers of controlled substances in Florida to also be dispensers of them, which made it relatively simple and easy for this criminal activity to take place. Additionally, Florida was a bit "late to the game" in implementing a state-funded Prescription Drug Monitoring Program (PDMP) to track prescribing patterns and identify people who sought prescriptions for opioids from multiple clinicians. Since then, things have changed in Florida, including legislation and law enforcement that directly targeted "pill mills," implementing a ban on clinic and clinician dispensing of controlled substances, and limits on quantities of medication which could be prescribed at one time. Reports of clinicians being identified and charged by the DEA for running pill mills still occur, but with a lower frequency than before. But many say that the "perfect storm" of identifying pain as a vital sign and a mandate to treat people with pain proved to be fertile ground for criminal activity, and created an immeasurable number of people who became addicted to opioids, fueling the nation's overdose epidemic.

Congress played a role in supporting the designation of pain as the 5th vital sign as well. Even though many may not remember it, in 2000, Congress voted to amend the Controlled Substances Act (CSA) of 1970, which created the scheduling of controlled substances, with the *Pain Relief Promotion act of 2000* [9]. This amended the CSA with the intention that there would be "*a new emphasis on pain and palliative care*" and to amended the CSA "*to declare that, for that Act (the CSA) and any implementing regulations, alleviating pain or discomfort in the usual course of professional practice is a legitimate medical purpose for the dispensing, distributing, or administering of a controlled substance that is consistent with public health and safety, even if it may increase the risk of death*." This act also designated January 1, 2001, as the beginning of the "*Decade of Pain Control and Research.*"

This is in no way a comprehensive analysis of all the stakeholders who have been or continue to be "blamed" for pain being designated the 5th vital sign and what followed, but it does provide a sampling of what was and has been happening with respect to this. What I am baffled by is that **what was completely missing from any of the blaming that was going on was the issue of whether the use of opioid analgesics to treat pain was _ethical or not_**. In most instances, there was no mention of ethics at all, only actions based on *re*action to the increased incidence of opioid-related overdoses and overdose fatalities.

The Overdose Epidemic

Regardless of how the overdose epidemic is conceptualized, according to the CDC at the time of this writing, approximately **187 people die every day in the United States from an opioid-related overdose** [10].

The terms "**opioid epidemic**" and "**overdose epidemic**" are unfortunately often used interchangeably by many stakeholders and media outlets. In many people's opinions, they are one and the same. With the CDC reporting that approximately 75% of heroin users stating that their first substance of nonmedical use was a prescription opioid, it seemed to connect the dots for many that increased opioid prescribing fueled the epidemic of overdoses and overdose fatalities. The blame for the epidemic lay squarely on the shoulders of all who embraced pain as the 5th vital sign, those who responded with a prescription for an opioid analgesic (e.g., frontline practitioners), those who promoted their use (opioid pharmaceutical manufacturers), and those whose criminal activity contributed to their illicit distribution and use.

The CDC refers to the "opioid epidemic" or the pattern of opioid-related overdose deaths as occurring in **three distinct "waves"** [10]. **The "first wave"** refers to the increased number of opioid-related overdose deaths between 1999 and 2010, which mainly involved fatalities associated with prescription opioids. It is not difficult to see a strong correlation between graphs that depict an increase in opioid prescribing related to pain being designated the 5th vital sign and an increase in opioid-related deaths; they essentially mirror each other. **The "second wave"** refers to the period between 2010 and 2013, with a dramatic increase in heroin-related overdose deaths, and the reformulation of Oxycontin® to an abuse-deterrent formulation. **The "third wave"** refers to the period from 2013 on, where there was (and still is) a dramatic increase in synthetic opioid-related (e.g., fentanyl and its analogues) overdose deaths. Recently, many have started to also refer to a **"fourth wave"** [11], which refers to the recent increased incidence of combined stimulant/opioid-related overdose deaths. It is possible that a **"5th wave"** is beginning right now with respect to the number of increasing overdoses of fentanyl and a drug named xylazine, a veterinary sedative, but that remains to be seen.

Explanations for the abovementioned "waves" are many. **With respect to the "first wave,"** it is hard to not attribute causality between the increased prescribing of opioids to treat the newly designated "vital sign." In fact, it might be wrong *not* to attribute causality. As mentioned earlier, there certainly was no shortage of stakeholders who to some degree participated in the "opiophilia" which was taking place at the time. Many like to assign the responsibility based on their own views, including blaming "big bad pharma," clinicians who were claiming to be experts but essentially "drug pushers" who were running pill mills, [12] and clinicians who were just naively trying to do what they could to treat people who complained of pain that was not successfully treated with other means. Nora Volkow, the Director of the National Institute on Drug Abuse (NIDA), wrote a research letter [13] to the *Journal of the American Medical Association* in 2011 that reported the results of an examination of the characteristics of opioid prescribers who wrote opioid prescriptions in 2009 to help to better understand prescribing practices and possible contributors to the high rate of nonmedical opioid analgesic use. This report identified that for patients over age 18, opioid prescriptions were written 43% of the time by Primary Care Physicians (General Practitioners, Family Medicine Physicians, Internal Medicine Physicians)—frontline practitioners, followed by Dentists in a distant second place. In this letter, Dr. Volkow also made two other important comments. First, that most nonmedical users *"reported that they obtained opioid prescriptions on their own or were given the medications from friends and relatives who had been prescribed opioids."* Second, that *"Our conclusions are limited because causal links with opioid diversion and abuse cannot be drawn from prescribing practices alone, and our analysis cannot account for illegal prescriptions."* **One thing that may have been overlooked is whether the** *patients who were prescribed opioids for pain were the ones who were dying* **during the "first wave" of the "opioid epidemic."** Things that are frequently overlooked include the fact that a sizable portion of nonmedical users of opioids (including heroin, fentanyl, etc.) *do* report that prescription opioids were indeed their first substance of nonmedical use. **But were they patients with pain or did they obtain the opioids from family members and friends?** The latter was (and still is) true most of the time, but that does not mean the former did not occur. Patients who were indiscriminately prescribed opioids in some cases did become addicted and/or did use them in ways other than directed. However the strongest connection between liberal prescribing of opioids to treat pain as the 5th vital sign in patients with pain and opioid-related overdose and overdose fatalities may well be that when opioids were prescribed, there was virtually often no discussion with patients about how they should be stored, that it was (and is) illegal for a patient to share a controlled substance like an opioid with *anyone else*, and that any opioids should be disposed of appropriately when they were no longer needed for the pain for which they were prescribed. It is fair to say that in the situation where someone who was prescribed an opioid analgesic and no longer needed it, that it was typical behavior then (and still is) for it to be saved for future use by the patient or other member of the household—*just in case*. This means that there might have been some amount of opioid that was stored in a medicine cabinet or some other easily accessible location in reserve, just waiting for someone to take some or all of it for nonmedical reasons. I consider this to be **an educational failing**, and something which may have contributed significantly to the "first wave." At the time, there was no shortage of mention in opioid prescribing guidelines that healthcare professional education and education of future healthcare professionals was a critical effort needed to help mitigate the overdose epidemic. It just did not often happen with respect to some simple things which could have been done to ensure responsibility of both prescriber and patient with respect to making sure that opioids were not accessible to others, were not be shared with others, and were disposed of when no longer needed. There were some efforts made by opioid manufacturers, such as creating special "lock boxes," which did not succeed to any significant degree in part because they were either too complicated, costly, or confusing. **A simple set of instructions—do not share, store safely, and get rid of the opioid when the pain improved and the opioid was no longer needed, may have had a better chance of success.** This could have been "baked into" standard clinician practices just like instructions that are given when anticoagulation therapy is initiated. Simple and to the point, and relatively easy to communicate and understand. It just did not happen, and still largely does even not happen today in most cases. Couple this with the fact that when the abovementioned Primary Care Physicians were prescribing those opioids during that "first wave," they were often making sure to prescribe a larger supply than likely needed to make sure that the patient would be "covered" during off-hours, weekends, etc., without instructions about disposal, without instructions about the illegality of sharing, and without instructions about the hazards associated with nonmedical use.

Additionally, **another educational failing** was that during this period of "liberal" opioid prescribing, clinicians were not taught about the importance of inquiring about the patient's past or present history of substance use, *and* the past or present history of substance use of other members of the household, or people who might potentially have access to the prescribed opioids. Virtually every regulatory agency from the White House-based Office of National Drug Control Policy to the FDA recommended that one key piece to battling this "first wave" was education about the importance of inquiring about past or present substance use history, not through education provided by pharmaceutical companies in the form of continuing education, but through education during training about the basics of responsibilities for patients and prescribers when opioids were prescribed. From an ethical perspective, leaving this information out of the clinician-patient dialogue during the assessment process essentially means that informed consent had not taken place.

Strategic thinking related to this "first wave" really needed to focus on the fact that **in many cases, patients were *not* the people who were becoming addicted or portraying aberrant drug-related behaviors (e.g., nonmedical use).** In many cases, the people dying in this "first wave" were people to whom the opioid was not prescribed, but who had obtained it from leftover or unsecured stores of opioids that had been prescribed. This was largely *not* a situation where the prescription opioids were "falling off the truck" or being stolen from pharmacies at gunpoint. It was a situation where they were being taken from sources which in many cases could be traced to a valid prescription. The lack of clarity and distinction about whether the "first wave" actually referred to patients who were prescribed an opioid for a valid pain complaint, non-patients who obtained an opioid from a diverted channel of distribution, or both, existed during this "first wave" and continues to exist today, with unclear messaging that implies that patients who were/are prescribed opioids for pain-related complaints were/are the people who were often succumbing to the opioid-related overdoses. It seems as if the moment the overdose (or "opioid") epidemic is mentioned, most believe that this is the result of over-prescribing an opioid to a patient with pain. There is *no question* that addiction and other aberrant behaviors do occur in patients who have been prescribed an opioid analgesic, in some cases with disastrous consequences. *There is also no question* that when an opioid is introduced into a household with members at "increased risk," that negative consequences may be more likely to occur related to those opioids. Additionally, something else that is often not discussed is the frequency with which someone who suffers an overdose or overdose fatality only has an opioid in their system responsible for the overdose. It is frequently reported that rarely is an opioid-related overdose or overdose fatality due to an opioid alone. In many cases, there are other substances in the person's system including an opioid, but those fatalities are commonly labeled as an "opioid-related" overdose, instead of a multisubstance event. Further, even though illicit substances are often responsible for the overdoses (which we will see in the "third wave"), such as heroin and fentanyl which are indeed opioids, it is often a de facto conclusion that the opioid overdoses involved prescribed opioids.

It is indisputable that clinicians who utilized opioids to treat pain during this "first wave" had an ethical responsibility to do many things to help mitigate the ensuing opioid epidemic while attempting to treat pain more effectively. This included an **evaluation risk of likelihood of addiction or potential for portraying aberrant drug-related behaviors**, to **perform a risk/benefit analysis that considered not only patient-level risk, but also risk to other members of the household**, to **convey a sense of responsibility** when opioids were prescribed, including safe storage and disposal, and to **warn patients about potential hazards associated with taking other medications which could potentially increase the adverse effect profile of an opioid** (including another prescribed or unprescribed opioid). Although most of these may seem like common-sense strategies, a coordinated effort through reinforced education could have possibly gone a long way toward helping clinicians at the time to negotiate the need (and mandate) to treat someone's pain, and to utilize opioid analgesics safely and effectively when indicated.

The "second wave" of opioid-related overdose deaths is considered by the CDC to have started in 2010 [10]. At this point in time, there was a dramatic uptick of heroin-related overdose fatalities. There are many things that may have contributed to this shift. Among them are the fact that heroin started to become significantly less expensive than prescription pain medications like oxycodone, which made it more attractive and more affordable as a substance of nonmedical use. Additionally, mandates were starting to trickle down from regulatory agencies like the White House Office of National Drug Control Policy (ONDCP) about the need to combat the rising tide of opioid overdose fatalities. In 2011, the ONDCP on behalf of the White House released a strategic plan titled *Epidemic: Responding to America's Prescription Drug Abuse Crisis* [14]. **This plan had four strategic "pillars."** The **first pillar** was **education of the public** about the dangers of nonmedical use of prescription pain medications like opioids, and **education of *all* healthcare-related professionals** about a multitude of related topics including appropriate prescribing, dispensing, and prevention of diversion, adverse effects, and addiction. This education was to be coordinated and provided by a multitude of agencies involved in healthcare administration and policy including the Food and Drug Administration, the Drug Enforcement Administration, the Centers for Disease Control and Prevention, and the Veteran's Health Administration to name a few. The **second pillar** was encouraging the use of Prescription Drug Monitoring Programs (PDMPs) to detect and prevent diversion and nonmedical use in all 50 states (not all states at this time had a PDMP). The **third pillar** was devoted to **proper medication disposal**, noting that "*a large source of the problem [the opioid epidemic] is a direct result of what is in Americans' medicine cabinets.*" It was noted that a 2009 Substance Abuse and Mental Health Administration found "**that over 70 percent of people who used prescription pain relievers non-medically got them from friends or relatives, while approximately 5 percent got them from a drug dealer or from the Internet.**" The plan suggested implementing more drug take-back events and facilitating disposal of unused and no-longer-needed opioid medications. Lastly, the **fourth pillar** of this plan was directed toward the role of law enforcement in helping to combat the illegitimate activities of "pill mills."

The coordinated educational efforts of the first pillar did not happen. In many cases, there were educational initiatives that were implemented, such as the Food and Drug Administration's Risk Evaluation and Mitigation Strategies (REMS), but undergraduate training programs were left out of the scope of the REMS, and in most cases this education was voluntary, time-consuming, and not widely embraced by most practicing clinicians, possibly due to time and resource constraints. In some cases, there were competing REMS opioid educational programs which further confused clinicians about which program was best to participate in, which might be more comprehensive, etc. With respect to PDMPs, reports have been mixed with respect to their efficacy, ability to share data across state lines, and their overall success in helping to stem the tide of overdose deaths. With respect to drug disposal, there are a few states that now have drug disposal containers located at every local police station (such as Florida), while others have one or two "national drug take-back days" which are often relatively poorly promoted, leaving public awareness relatively low. With respect to the role of law enforcement and its role in combatting illegitimate prescribing, there has been a relatively large degree of success; the prevalence of "pill mills" is much lower today than in the past.

But something else also contributed to this "second wave" and the move toward heroin-related overdoses. It is reasonable to say that between 2000 and 2010, during the first wave of the overdose crisis, Oxycontin® was considered by many to be the "poster child" of opioid analgesics used for nonmedical purposes. It was *the* most misused opioid of choice for many nonmedical users for several reasons, including its potency and ease of delivery by commonly desired alternative routes (alternative to oral ingestion or swallowing) of administration which included snorting a crushed pill, or injecting a melted or dissolved and extracted pill. Oxycontin provided users with a significant "bang for the buck" based on its cost, ease of availability, and perceived level of "safety" because it was pharmaceutical grade, and perceived to be safer than street-level drugs which could potentially be tainted with contaminants and not "pure." In response to a growing sense that it was significantly contributing to the overdose crisis, the manufacturer of Oxycontin®, Purdue Pharmaceuticals, applied to the FDA for permission to reformulate the drug to an abuse-deterrent formulation, which would theoretically make it more difficult for nonmedical users to crush or snort, or melt/extract, or inject, without needing to supply any other additional information to the FDA, since the drug had already been approved by the FDA in its non-abuse-deterrent form. The FDA approved the new formulation, and the newly approved and "reformulated" version of Oxycontin® became commercially available on August 9, 2010, and production of the former non-abuse-deterrent version ceased. The effect that this likely had on substance users was that to a certain degree, the "new" Oxycontin® was less "attractive" to users because of more hurdles to snort or inject it, and the increased street cost of this new formulation. This made heroin more "attractive." This likely inadvertently played a key role in the "second wave." In summary, it appears that at the time, heroin assumed a higher place on the desirability list for nonmedical users than Oxycontin® and other prescription opioid analgesics. There was a point in time in 2011 when oxymorphone was considered by some to be the "new" Oxycontin® for nonmedical users, with a number of mainstream media articles labeling it as the new prescription pain drug of choice for substance users in light of the reformulated Oxycontin®, but heroin was the most frequent alternative with a steady increase of heroin-related overdoses through 2015.

In 2013, the **"third wave"** of opioid-related overdoses is considered to have begun. At this time, heroin overdoses were still on a steady rise, but something new that had been relatively under the radar started to emerge—**synthetic opioids**. These opioids were quite "attractive" as they could be manufactured relatively inexpensively, easily, and virtually anywhere if drug dealers were able to obtain the necessary ingredients, which were readily available from a number of illicit sources including the Dark Web. The "poster child" for these synthetic opioids was **fentanyl**, a potent opioid that is approximately 100 times more potent than morphine. Fentanyl was originally developed to be used as an anesthetic agent to be used by Anesthesiology personnel, in a controlled setting with resuscitative equipment readily available because of its increased potential for significant respiratory depression due to its potency. Its safety profile was incredibly high, with the amount needed to be lethal by poisoning being somewhere between 20,000–50,000 times the therapeutically effective dose—in the proper hands. Outside of a controlled setting, fentanyl has the potential to be quite dangerous, because it could cause respiratory arrest quickly, **leading to death**. A problem was that fentanyl provided experienced opioid users with a "better high," either alone or in combination with other drugs, sometimes including heroin. Just adding the smallest amount of fentanyl to heroin made it significantly more potent, more "attractive" to substance users, and significantly more deadly. It did not take long for fentanyl and other "sibling compounds" of fentanyl (analogues such as carfentanil) to become the leading cause of opioid-related overdoses and overdose deaths. It is worth noting that carfentanil, typically used as a large animal (e.g., elephant) anesthetic agent, is 100 times more potent than fentanyl, making it 10,000 times more potent than morphine. In 2015, synthetic opioid-related deaths soared past heroin and commonly prescribed opioid-related deaths. The graphic display of the third wave has been almost a straight vertical line upwards which continues to increase today.

Experienced nonmedical drug users are not the only people who have been dying of overdoses because of fentanyl. Naïve nonmedical users, such as teenagers trying drugs for the first time, are being exposed to fentanyl and its analogues more frequently because of consuming counterfeit pills that look genuine, but have been tainted with fentanyl, or using drugs like marijuana or cocaine which has been tainted with fentanyl or its analogues. **Fentanyl and other synthetic opioid-related overdoses now dominate** opioid-related fatalities around the United States and other parts of the world.

There is now speculation of the existence of a "**fourth wave**" of overdose deaths [11] which refers to overdose fatalities which are characterized as involving stimulants like methamphetamine along with or without a synthetic opioid like fentanyl. This "wave" appears to be characterized by polysubstance nonmedical use, and it remains to be seen what might be effective in terms of mitigating this new tide of drug-related fatalities, because naloxone has no effect on methamphetamines.

Along with the timelining of opioid-related overdoses identified by the CDC, there have been many approaches that have been tried from a regulatory perspective to thwart the steady increase in overdoses and overdose fatalities, and they have been mentioned in other areas of this book with respect to the opioid epidemic. They include but are not limited to the U.S. Food and Drug Administration Risk Evaluation and Mitigation Strategies (REMS) for opioid analgesics, the development of state managed Prescription Drug Monitoring Program databases, the encouragement of clinicians to consider the appropriateness of co-prescribing naloxone to individuals being treated with opioid therapy at increased risk for respiratory depression, increasing access to naloxone to people who use opioids nonmedically, shutting down "pill mills," and prosecuting nefarious prescribers. Additionally, a number of harm reduction strategies have been expolored, including needle exchange programs, safe injection sites, and community-level naloxone distribution at no cost.

One regulatory approach to mitigating the "opioid epidemic" **has superseded all the others—decreasing the number of opioids prescribed and the number of prescriptions written. Regulators went "all in" with respect to a strategy that if fewer opioids were prescribed, there would be fewer opioid-related overdoses and overdose fatalities**. As mentioned previously, when the **CDC released its opioid guidelines in 2016**, one of the most famous (and most contentious) parts of the guidelines was the recommended ceiling of morphine milligram equivalents of opioid prescribed daily. In essence, the message sent was that unless the clinician was an expert with more training (e.g., pain specialist), the recommendations were that these ceilings should be adhered to, or there should be documentation in the medical record as to why higher doses of opioids above the ceiling were necessary. In many cases, state medical boards incorporated these dosing restrictions into their opioid prescribing guidelines, and the Drug Enforcement Administration (DEA) along with the state medical boards began to review PDMP data to not only identify patients who were seeking prescriptions from multiple providers, but to identify clinicians who were found to be outside of "acceptable" prescribing patterns compared to similar clinicians of the same discipline. In other words, a primary care clinician who prescribed opioids outside of these recommended ceiling doses could potentially face regulatory scrutiny from the DEA, the state medical board, or both. The effect was chilling, in that many clinicians felt that one of two things needed to happen in order for them to avoid this regulatory scrutiny: either forcibly taper patients who were being prescribed more than the ceiling dose limit, or stop writing prescriptions for opioids altogether. In both cases, the effect left some bona fide pain patients who relied on opioids to effectively manage their pain to find somewhere else to go for a prescription, which was challenging and, in some cases, not possible. The emphasis was to have less opioids available to people who might use them nonmedically and overdose from them. Haphazard attempts at clinician education were made, but not in a coordinated manner. **The DEA also implemented restrictions on quantities of opioids that could be manufactured and distributed**, essentially making less opioids available to be prescribed. Healthcare systems implemented restrictions on opioid prescribing in a variety of ways, including in some cases prohibiting prescription of opioids for all but postoperative patients.

By the time it started to become apparent that there was a possibility that these collective efforts were possibly leading to "misapplication" by clinicians and resulting in unintended, negative consequences to patients with pain as a direct result of the implementation of the 2016 CDC guidelines [15], artificially created medication shortages by the DEA manufacturing restrictions, and ultimately decreased access of opioids to patients who needed them to adequately control their pain, in some ways, the damage had been done. Clinicians "received the message" that opioids were not the best choice of pain treatment for most patients, and that nonopioid alternatives were better, regardless of their efficacy, availability, or reimbursement. Regulators uniformly believed that a **decrease in opioid prescribing by healthcare professionals was going to solve the "opioid epidemic."** Regardless of whether the majority of overdoses were resulting from illicit opioids or not, the thinking was that what needed to happen was less prescribing of opioid analgesics.

In September of 2021, the American Medical Association released a report titled *Physicians' actions to help end the nation's drug-related overdose and death epidemic —and what still needs to be done* [16]. **The report began by detailing that as of 2021, "***opioid prescriptions decreased for the 10th consecutive year, but [overdose] deaths continued to increase. It's time to change course.***"** The report stated that there was a continuing increase in drug-related mortality (approximately 94,134 overdose deaths) despite a 44.4% decrease in opioid prescriptions between 2011 and 2021, a significant increase in PDMP utilization, and increased use of buprenorphine use for people with substance use disorder over the same period of time. In 2022, the AMA updated this report [17], reflecting that opioid prescribing continued a downward trend (46.4% decrease in opioid prescriptions between 2012–2021) while overdose and deaths related to illicitly manufactured fentanyl, methamphetamine, and cocaine continued to increase (approximately 107,521 overdose deaths in 2021). In both reports, the AMA called for multiple efforts including harm reduction strategies, increased access to patients in need of substance use treatment, and standardization of data to better identify populations at risk, while maintaining access to opioids and nonopioids for those with pain in need, especially underserved and disparate patient populations.

These two AMA reports illustrated that the "silver-bullet" strategy of solely decreasing the number of opioid prescriptions written was not solving the **overdose epidemic**. Just by virtue that in most of the mainstream media, regulatory agency briefings, and many scientific publications that the overdose epidemic is still referred to as the "opioid epidemic," which invokes the thought that the epidemic is mostly related to prescription opioids signals to me that things may be getting "lost in the shuffle" and that intentions might be confused. It is still quite common today to see something published or written about drug-related fatalities with a stock photo of a prescription pain pill accompanying its narrative. Questions in my mind involve what the role of healthcare professionals was and is in terms of mitigating overdoses and overdose fatalities which involve illicit substances like synthetic opioids (i.e., fentanyl and its analogues). It seemed to me over the course of the past 24 years that **education was *and continues to be* critical**, and that if there are significant numbers of people as young as age 12 who are being exposed to these substances through unhealthy or nonmedical use, education starting prior to this age would be considered an appropriate and important thing to do. This does not negate the fact that appropriate prescribing practices, risk mitigation strategies, and careful monitoring need to be employed by prescribers. But it also means that these approaches need to work together in an educated fashion to make things safer, *without denying patients* who might be appropriate candidates for opioids as a component of their pain treatment.

There seems to be a lack of intentionality about the way to deal with the rising number of overdose fatalities, beyond a reactive, "whack a mole" approach. Certainly, there is a desire to stop the number of people who succumb to intentional or unintentional drug-related deaths and there should be. But the simple things seem to have been overlooked and lines have become blurry. For example, it is not uncommon for people to refer to the fentanyl that has become significantly responsible for most of the overdose deaths as "*illicit* fentanyl." In my opinion, this implies that the fentanyl being manufactured by drug dealers is in some ways more dangerous than pharmaceutical grade fentanyl—it is not. In fact, illicitly manufactured fentanyl is often equivalent to pharmaceutical grade fentanyl. Fentanyl, as mentioned previously, is a very potent opioid, and whether or not it is illicitly manufactured is not really the issue. The issue is that a powerful agent like fentanyl is quite dangerous to anyone who is exposed to it in the absence of someone with expertise in managing airways with resuscitative equipment available in all but the most limited situations, such as patients who are prescribed it for intractable pain in the variety of available formulations.

The fact that counterfeit pills and other illicit drugs are being tainted with fentanyl should invoke public awareness campaigns related to caution and prevention. When opioid analgesics are prescribed, it should be as common to discuss with patients the importance of safe storage, proper disposal, and the unlawfulness of sharing them with *anyone* as discussing the potential dangers associated with anticoagulant therapy when those medications are prescribed. From an ethical perspective, this information should be included as part of the informed consent process.

As mentioned many times throughout the course of this book, memories seem to be short with respect to the role of communication and education in promoting prevention of overdoses and overdose fatalities. A case in point was illustrated well in the state of Utah in 2009, with its Prescription Pain Medication Program [18]. In 2007, the **Utah State Legislature passed a Bill, HB-137** to combat deaths and other harms associated with prescription opioids used to treat people with chronic pain. At the time, Utah was one of the first states (possibly *the first*) to see the number of annual drug-related overdose fatalities outnumber motor vehicle-related fatalities. This bill established a two-year program with the goals of: **reducing the number of deaths resulting from prescription medications by 15% by educating providers, patients, insurers, and the public, better understanding of deaths related to prescription pain medications and understanding of prescribing patterns and other risk factors that increased risk of death, and to provide recommendations about the use of the PDMP to help identify patients at increased risk and prevent deaths associated with prescription pain medications.**

This program utilized a multipronged approach to aggressive "academic detailing" or education [19] to the abovementioned stakeholders about safe prescribing practices and responsible behaviors of individuals to whom opioids were prescribed. The results of this two-year program included a significant reduction in prescription drug-related deaths (~14%), identification of and understanding of specific predisposing risk factors for potential for overdose death, such as being unemployed, obese, female, and depressed, and a set of opioid prescribing clinical guidelines for clinicians practicing in the state of Utah. This proved the hypothesis that **education of stakeholders could potentially make a positive difference**. At the time, it was estimated that it would take about 10 years of aggressive educational efforts for a program like this to make a sustainable and durable difference. Unfortunately, this program was not refunded by the state of Utah, and two years later, the ground that was gained had been lost in terms of overdose deaths related to prescription pain medications. Even though the success and nature of this aggressive educational program was well documented in the scientific literature, it was not replicated by other states and their departments of health and touted as a significant and important approach to maintaining access and mitigating risk.

Researchers in the Utah program noted five key takeaways, which in my opinion still are true today. First, that collaboration with local healthcare organizations and their staff was essential in **helping entire clinics understand the epidemic and engage in prevention.** Second, that it was important to **adapt processes so they work best for clinicians; not to change their behaviors, but to complement them**. Third, that **ease of access to the PDMP** and time and resources required to access the PDMP were key factors determining its overall utility. Fourth, that **coordinated efforts between researchers and regulatory officials** increased the likelihood of better understanding and tailoring approaches towards the overdose epidemic. Lastly, the recommendation that **words and approaches matter**, and that intention to change behavior might have been better word smithed to something focused more on standardization of practices than changing behaviors.

Some valuable remnants of this project in Utah continue to live on, **with a website directed toward the public** to "know your script" https://knowyourscript.org/, an online educational resource that teaches patients their roles and responsibilities in asking questions, using prescribed medications properly, and avoiding risks. **This resource also focuses on the importance of preventive strategies,** including parents "having the talk" with children about risks of using drugs, educating and empowering them to ask questions, and to develop pro-social skills, being aware of social triggers such as divorce, depression, and bullying which could potentially predispose children to exhibiting "risky" behaviors and increasing the likelihood of addiction. The Utah opioid prescribing guidelines are among the most practical and logical I have seen. They could have been a boilerplate for other state departments of health to adopt and employ. It is worthy to reemphasize that this project in Utah took place **in 2009**.

The word "**poison**" can have several meanings. Typically, as a noun, it refers to "a substance that through its chemical action usually kills, injures, or impairs an organism." [20] The common inferred implication is that there is some type of toxicity and resulting organ damage, which may be permanent or temporary depending on the substance to which one is exposed. For example, the over-the-counter medication acetaminophen is hepatotoxic in large enough quantities (i.e., overdose) which can cause permanent liver damage and liver failure [21]. **It *is* possible to suffer from acetaminophen poisoning. Nonsteroidal anti-inflammatory drugs, which are also widely available both over-the-counter and by prescription, have also been reported to be acutely toxic** if taken in large enough quantities (i.e., overdose), resulting in a number of serious sequelae including convulsions, metabolic acidosis, coma, and acute renal failure [22].

The overdose epidemic in the context of opioid substances is most often <u>*not*</u> the result of "poisoning" in a traditional sense, despite the very frequent use of the term opioid poisoning by the media, regulatory agencies, and even in the scientific literature. **The fatalities associated with opioid overdoses are uniformly associated with one the most serious adverse effects of opioids—respiratory depression.**

Words matter and **using the term "opioid poisoning" instead of opioid overdose implies that there has been some type of toxicity or organ damage-like event that has taken place, not the consequence of adverse effects.** Opioids may cause people to fall and become injured, they may cause people to lose consciousness or become cognitively impaired, and in the case of synthetic opioids like fentanyl, they *will* cause someone to stop breathing, possibly resulting in a fatal outcome. That being said, although toxicity from a drug like fentanyl *is* theoretically possible, as mentioned earlier in this chapter, the amount of fentanyl needed to actually be poisonous or toxic is estimated to be somewhere between 20,000 and 50,000 times the therapeutic dose, which makes the likelihood of fentanyl 'poisoning' highly unlikely because the person is likely to die as a result of respiratory arrest long before toxicity occurs. It is possible that the parties using the term "opioid poisoning" are attempting to use terminology which lay people will better understand, but it is also possible and likely that the term may be misunderstood. I have seen overdose and poisoning used interchangeably many times in the past 24 years, and in the spirit of informed consent, I believe that everyone has a responsibility to be accurate with respect to the differences between the two situations.

This phenomenon of inaccurate nomenclature has also impacted naloxone, with **naloxone often being referred to by many as an "antidote"** to an "opioid poisoning." **The classical definition of antidote is "a remedy to counteract the effects of a poison."** In the context of a respiratory arrest or respiratory depressive episode created by a relative overdose of opioids, naloxone *is* a **reversal agent**, or opioid antagonist, which acts competitively to counteract the respiratory or cognitive effect of the opioid, as well as its analgesic effect. But **naloxone has no action related to the treatment of opioid toxicity**, *if* it were to exist in a given situation. The reason that this is so important in the context of the overdose epidemic, is that inaccuracy of the nomenclature used in these contexts is often related to educational deficits, which may then lead to miscommunication, misunderstanding, unrealistic expectations, and unethical treatment of people with pain.

Ethics and Opioid Prescribing

Controversy regarding the ethics of using opioids to treat chronic pain has existed since 2000, when pain was designated the 5th vital sign and is complicated with respect to the overdose epidemic. Specifically, the controversy often surrounds the question of the needs and desires of the patient versus the needs or potential danger not only to the patient, but to the community and to society.

In 2010, Ballantyne and Fleisher published an article [23] about ethical issues when prescribing opioid analgesics for the treatment of chronic pain. They discussed a shift from paternalistic care of patients to shared decision-making in the context of utilizing opioids to treat people with chronic pain, without necessarily considering the potential addictive nature of opioids for the sake of patient satisfaction. This article stressed that if the ethical mandate of benevolence (presumably beneficence) is a main driver for the clinician, it is also important to consider circumstances where opioid analgesic therapy may or may not be beneficial, and, in some cases, be detrimental. Not only detrimental to the individual patient, but also detrimental to society in terms of abuse, misuse, and opioid-related fatalities. They pose the question as to *"whether patients' wishes should override costs to society."* Further, these authors state *"In the United States, the ethos is that patients' choices should be respected, regardless of cost to society. In the opioid debate, the cost to society is the cost of abuse and misuse. If the clinician sees merit in opioid therapy for an individual patient, then traditional values of duty to patient apply. But for the patient who claims a right to treatment that is not agreed upon, in that case the clinician must surely step outside the bounds of the therapeutic bond and consider the broader consequences to society of opioids provided solely on the basis of demand. After all, when clinicians fail to control abuse and misuse, the regulatory authorities step in, and the freedom to prescribe is constrained, possibly leading back along the path to unnecessary suffering."* They concluded by stating *"there will be conditions such as those posited here, that strongly suggest that opioid treatment is not suitable, and should be denied, even when the patient demands it, or claims satisfaction."*

Five years later, in 2015, Cohen and Jangro [24] published an article that was in part a response to Ballantyne and Fleisher's abovementioned article, and also in part to call attention to a need for progress to be made in the medical community with respect to using ethics to guide clinical decision-making with respect to the use of opioid analgesic therapy in chronic (noncancer) pain. These authors differed in their opinion of the mandate to alleviated pain and associated suffering of the individual, pointing out that a significant percentage of people with cancer-related and noncancer related pain were being left untreated or under-treated as a result of stigmatization of opioid therapy. Cohen and Jangro posited that because of the lack of substantial scientific evidence about the benefits of long-term opioid therapy (referring to it as "data-thin"), the ethical approach to using opioid therapy for chronic pain treatment rested in being patient-centered and not population-based, focusing on autonomy, shared decision-making, mutual (clinician/patient) goal-setting, attention to biopsychosocial factors, and improved quality of life. They proposed

six steps to the ethical use of opioid therapy: **capturing the patient's narrative** about how pain affects their life, **making a diagnosis or at least attempting to identify the pathophysiological basis** for the patient's pain, **setting goals that are collaborative and individualized** to the patient's needs, **measuring progress or regress** with respect to the implemented treatment plan (including opioid therapy), **replacing accomplished goals with "subgoals,"** and lastly, making sure to **revisit clinical decisions regarding opioid therapy in the face of new clinically relevant scientific data** as it becomes available.

These two articles provide a representative sample of the debates about opioid analgesic therapy that have taken place over the past 24 years. It has been and continues to be a complex issue, with few mentions that ethics should be what ultimately guides clinical decisions about opioid analgesic therapy, mitigatigating societal risk, and helping to tame the overdose epidemic which continues to worsen each year.

References

1. National Capital Poison Center. The opioid pendulum: balancing its risks and benefits. https://www.poison.org/articles/the-opioid-pendulum-opioid-risks-and-benefits-182. Accessed 18 July 2023.
2. Chou R, Fanciullo GJ, Fine PG, Adler JA, Ballantyne JC, Davies P, Donovan MI, Fishbain DA, Foley KM, Fudin J, Gilson AM, Kelter A, Mauskop A, O'Connor PG, Passik SD, Pasternak GW, Portenoy RK, Rich BA, Roberts RG, Todd KH, Miaskowski C. American Pain Society-American Academy of Pain Medicine Opioids Guidelines Panel. Clinical guidelines for the use of chronic opioid therapy in chronic noncancer pain. J Pain. 2009 Feb;10(2):113–30.
3. U.S. Senate Homeland Security & Governmental Affairs Committee, Ranking Member's Office. Fueling an epidemic: exposing the financial ties between Opioid Manufacturers and Third Party Advocacy Groups. https://www.hsgac.senate.gov/wp-content/uploads/imo/media/doc/REPORT-Fueling%20an%20Epidemic-Exposing%20the%20Financial%20Ties%20Between%20Opioid%20Manufacturers%20and%20Third%20Party%20Advocacy%20Groups.pdf. Accessed 21 July 2023.
4. The Veterans Health Administration. TAKE 5: pain: the 5th vital sign. https://www.google.com/url?sa=t&rct=j&q=&esrc=s&source=web&cd=&cad=rja&uact=8&ved=2ahUKEwje0KbxtqCAAxXKEFkFHZqeBtAQFnoECA8QAQ&url=https%3A%2F%2Fwww.va.gov%2Fpainmanagement%2Fdocs%2Ftoolkit.pdf&usg=AOvVaw3XBh3AxY6fpKaMA3rXNwNI&opi=89978449. Accessed 21 July 2023.
5. Baker DW. History of the Joint Commission's pain standards: lessons for Today's prescription opioid epidemic. JAMA. 2017;317(11):1117–8.
6. Jones MR, Viswanath O, Peck J, Kaye AD, Gill JS, Simopoulos TT. A brief history of the opioid epidemic and strategies for pain medicine. Pain Ther. 2018;7(1):13–21.
7. Clark K, Rogers H. Corrupting influence: Purdue the WHO. Exposing dangerous opioid manufacturer influence at the World Health Organization. May 22, 2019. Available at: https://katherineclark.house.gov/2019/5/clark-rogers-release-report-exposing-purdue-pharma-s-corrupting-influence-at-the-world-health-organization#:~:text=The%20report%20reveals%20that%20two,increase%20prescriptions%20and%20expand%20sales. Accessed 21 July 2023.
8. Spencer T. Florida "pill mills" were the "gas on the fire" of opioid crisis. Associated Press; 2019. Available at: https://apnews.com/article/0ced46b203864d8fa6b8fda6bd97b60e. Accessed 21 July 2023.

9. Representative Hyde, Henry J. H.R.2260—Pain Relief Promotion Act of 2000. Congress. gov. Available at https://www.congress.gov/bill/106th-congress/house-bill/2260. Accessed 25 July 2023.

10. Centers for Disease Control and Prevention. Understanding the epidemic. https://www.cdc.gov/opioids/basics/epidemic.html. Accessed 25 July 2023.

11. Jenkins RA. The fourth wave of the US opioid epidemic and its implications for the rural US: a federal perspective. Prev Med. 2021;152(Pt 2):106541.

12. Rosenberg T. When is a pain doctor a drug pusher? The New York Times, June 17, 2007.

13. Volkow ND, McLellan TA, Cotto JH, Karithanom M, Weiss SR. Characteristics of opioid prescriptions in 2009. JAMA. 2011;305(13):1299–301.

14. Executive Office of the President of the United States, President Barack Obama. Epidemic: responding to America's Prescription Drug Abuse Crisis. 2011. Available at: https://www.google.com/url?sa=t&rct=j&q=&esrc=s&source=web&cd=&cad=rja&uact=8&ved=2ahUKEwjm7KmooqqAAxUihIkEHavOBDAQFnoECBoQAQ&url=https%3A%2F%2Fobamawhitehouse.archives.gov%2Fsites%2Fdefault%2Ffiles%2Fondcp%2Fpolicy-and-research%2Frx_abuse_plan.pdf&usg=AOvVaw1dsCybhJt4LGGlgnUD5pOr&opi=89978449. Accessed 25 July 2023.

15. Dowell D, Haegerich TM, Chou R. CDC guideline for prescribing opioids for chronic pain – United States, 2016. MMWR Recomm Rep. 2016;65(1):1–49.

16. The American Medical Association. Physicians' actions to help end the nation's drug-related overdose and death epidemic—and what still needs to be done. 2021. https://end-overdose-epidemic.org/. Accessed 22 June 2023.

17. The American Medical Association. Physicians' actions to help end the nation's drug-related overdose and death epidemic—and what still needs to be done. 2022. https://end-overdose-epidemic.org/. Accessed 22 June 2023.

18. Utah Department of Health. HB-137 Final report: prescription pain medication program. February 19, 2009. Available at: https://www.google.com/url?sa=t&rct=j&q=&esrc=s&source=web&cd=&cad=rja&uact=8&ved=2ahUKEwiQoqPwqaqAAxWKE1kFHbbyAdgQFnoECAwQAQ&url=https%3A%2F%2Fhealth.utah.gov%2Fprescription%2Fpdf%2F2009final_programreport.pdf&usg=AOvVaw153f297T150doR7C4_AEX2&opi=89978449. Accessed 25 July 2023.

19. Cochella S, Bateman K. Provider detailing: an intervention to decrease prescription opioid deaths in Utah. Pain Med. 2011;12(Suppl 2):S73–6.

20. Definition of Poison. https://www.merriam-webster.com/dictionary/poison. Accessed 25 July 2023.

21. McNeil Consumer Healthcare. Guidelines for the management of acetaminophen overdose. Available at: https://www.google.com/url?sa=t&rct=j&q=&esrc=s&source=web&cd=&cad=rja&uact=8&ved=2ahUKEwill8WyrKqAAxWsmokEHTngC_MQFnoECA0QAQ&url=https%3A%2F%2Fwww.tylenolprofessional.com%2Fsites%2Ftylenol_hcp_us%2Ffiles%2Facetaminphen_overdose_treatment_info.pdf&usg=AOvVaw0OMQsygMLxehLxBRpS-_gI&opi=89978449. Accessed 25 July 2023.

22. Hunter LJ, Wood DM, Dargan PI. The patterns of toxicity and management of acute nonsteroidal anti-inflammatory drug (NSAID) overdose. Open Access Emerg Med. 2011;6(3):39–48.

23. Ballantyne JC, Fleisher LA. Ethical issues in opioid prescribing for chronic pain. Pain. 2010;148(3):365–7.

24. Cohen MJ, Jangro WC. A clinical ethics approach to opioid treatment of chronic noncancer pain. AMA J Ethics. 2015;17(6):521–9.

The Static Pendulum

16

Pain and Drugs: A Pendulum in Motion

Since 2000, there has been constant change with respect to pain and how it is managed, substance use, and the intersection and relationship between them. In many cases, these changes have been "reactive" in one way or another, in many cases in response to some type of stimulus, action, or demand for action.

When pain was designated as **the 5th vital sign** in 2000, presumably it was most likely with the intention of identifying people with pain who in many cases were either left untreated, undertreated, or ignored—a situation which was highly prevalent at the time. One "reaction" was to make pain assessment part of virtually all clinical encounters to give pain the attention it deserved. Depending on what you read, it is also possible that another motivation or "action" was part of a masterful marketing campaign by opioid manufacturers, the result of financial influence and lobbying efforts by those same manufacturers toward patient advocacy groups and/or professional organizations devoted to pain management, political lobbying by the opioid manufacturers who in some cases had significant financial influence, legislation by congress and the federal government, a mandate to improve the quality of care to people with pain from organizations like the Joint Commission, or some combination of all of the above or more "actions." Regardless of the specifics, there was a lot of activity devoted to bringing pain and its impact front and center, and ever since there has been a lot of "reaction" with respect to pain, the most recognizable reaction being making routine clinical assessments include a query about the presence or absence of pain and its rating on a numerical scale of 0–10 with 0 being no pain at all, and 10 being pain as bad as it could be. This was a major "swing of the pendulum" toward bringing attention to something that was considered to be plaguing a substantial percentage of the U.S. population. **Patients were empowered by pain advocacy groups to the fact that they had a "Bill of Rights" which demanded their pain to be assessed and treated.**

At the time, any type of pain was essentially considered to be the same for all patients with respect to its assessment and treatment. Pain was considered to be

© The Author(s), under exclusive license to Springer Nature Switzerland AG 2024   197
K. L. Zacharoff, P. Migdal, *Pain, Drugs, and Ethics*,
https://doi.org/10.1007/978-3-031-63018-7_16

a symptom that required the application of standard clinical paradigms that were familiar to all clinicians in practice or in training; identify the chief complaint (in this case pain complaint); perform physical, historical, and laboratory evaluations; and at a minimum, arrive at a differential diagnosis, communicate the presumptive diagnosis to the patient, formulate a treatment plan, implement that plan, and then reassess and follow-up as necessary. For patients with chronic pain (i.e., pain lasting 3 months duration or longer), if the follow-up revealed no presence of adverse effects related to the treatment plan with some degree of improvement in the numerical pain rating, the medical note would often include "continue current treatment" and the patient would be sent on their way, often with a prescription renewal for their pain medication, which in many cases, included or consisted solely of an opioid analgesic. What in fact made pain different from other medical conditions was that in many situations, the patient's pain ratings were subjective in nature, often eluded the ability to make a specific diagnosis which could be confirmed by testing and/or physical examination. In certain situations when there was clearly an acute injury which could clinically substantiate the pain-related complaint, especially in chronic pain situations, healing had already taken place and created doubts in the minds of clinicians about whether or not the patient was truly experiencing pain, sometimes leading to patients feeling stigmatized, shamed, embarrassed, and fearful of being labeled as malingerers.

At the time, the reactive pendulum certainly moved in the direction of identifying more people with pain, but unfortunately this was not in concert with increased education for clinicians and clinicians in training about best practices with respect to pain assessment and treatment. Clinicians often treated the pain rating as if it was hypertension or hyperglycemia because it was what they thought they were supposed to do. There was often no query about pain impact on function, overall quality of life, or communication leading to mutually-determined realistic goals and expectations of pain treatment. In the absence of a significant educational foundation about pain treatment, opioid analgesics were often the go-to treatment because virtually everyone expected "a prescription" to be the end-result of an office visit for a pain-related complaint. Pharmacologic treatment of pain which was unresponsive to over-the-counter medications like acetaminophen, nonsteroidal anti-inflammatory drugs, or other self-treatment home remedies was the norm, and opioid prescriptions were often the solution. Despite the fact that in the early 2000s, healthcare had already identified the ethical benefits of shared decision-making, in the world of pain management it was a situation where the clinician was frequently telling patients to "*Just do what I say*" and patients asking, "*Just tell me what to do to get rid of this pain.*" The need to query almost every patient about pain in the face of little or no education because it was now a "vital sign" seemed to create an atmosphere that consisted of decreased levels of communication, leading to decreased comprehension and increased confusion, a lack of informed consent, and increased opioid prescribing.

Attempts were made to provide much-needed guidance to frontline practitioners who in the course of their training had received little to no education about how to deal with this newly identified "vital sign" and to try to fill some of the glaring educational gaps involving opioid prescribing and the associated risk of aberrant drug-related behaviors or addiction. One prominent and well-respected example was a commentary published by Gourlay, Heit, and Almahrezi in 2005 [1]. These authors proposed that clinicians employ a "universal precautions" approach that be applied to *all* patients with chronic pain who were considered to be potential candidates for opioid analgesic treatment. They recommended 10 practical, logical steps which clinicians could relatively easily implement to improve safety, efficacy, and facilitate mitigation of risk related to aberrant behaviors, and the development of addictive disorders. Basically, the underlying premise was to consider *all* patients prescribed an opioid to be "at risk." Unfortunately, this commentary was published in the journal *Pain Medicine*, a publication which was not widely distributed to or frequently read by nonexpert, frontline practitioners. Most members of the pain community endorsed these relatively simple recommendations and considered them to be the foundation of good pain practice, but dissemination to those clinicians caring for most patients with pain were largely unaware of the "universal precautions approach," which might have had the potential to slow or even possibly reverse a "pendulum swing" toward avoiding opioids altogether because of the increased incidence of opioid-related overdoses and overdose fatalities.

In 2009, the American Pain Society and the American Academy of Pain Medicine jointly attempted once again to fill the void with respect to filling the educational voids of *"clinical skills and knowledge in both the principles of opioid prescribing and on the assessment and management of risks associated with opioid abuse, addiction, and diversion"* by publishing the results of a two-year evidence-based review by a number of multidisciplinary experts of the medical literature in the form of a set of opioid prescribing guidelines which were based on a scientific evidence rating. These guidelines were published in article titled *Clinical Guidelines for the Use of Chronic Opioid Therapy in Chronic Noncancer Pain* and published in both the *Journal of Pain* and the journal *Pain Medicine*, the respective scientific publications of these two professional pain organizations [2]. Similar to the abovementioned "universal precautions approach" to opioid prescribing by Gourlay and Heit et al, these guidelines were clinically practical and relevant to frontline clinical practitioners who were most in need of this type of guidance and recommendations. Once again, they were only disseminated in publications which were most likely to be read by expert-level clinicians, and did not reach most frontline practitioners. Ultimately, these guidelines fell out of favor because it was thought by many that since opioid manufacturers contributed significantly to both these organizations at the time, there was a distinct possibility of conflict of interest and pharma influence in the guideline messaging in a fashion that promoted opioid prescribing.

What followed these and other recommendations was a development of **several clinical dilemmas surrounding the utilization (or over-utilization) of opioid analgesics,** with numerous reactions related to these dilemmas. They included a number of other organizations that developed their own guidelines for safe and effective use of opioids to treat pain, a "pendulum swing" of the mainstream media toward decreased use of opioids and their "strong relationship to the overdose epidemic," and stigmatization directed toward clinicians who were either willing to continue to prescribe opioids relatively liberally, or on a long-term basis for patients with chronic pain. Educational programs were developed and released from a variety of different sources, including the FDA, the National Institue of Drug Abuse (NIDA), and the Federation of State Medical Boards, sometimes with competing and conflicting messaging about how opioids should be utilized to treat pain. Importantly, one of the most significant clinical dilemmas that reactively developed and continues to challenge clinicians today is fear in the minds of many clinicians of potential **regulatory scrutiny** if opioids were continued to be prescribed in their practices.

These dilemmas led to a frequent **lack of regimentation and consensus at a clinical level** about how and whether opioid analgesics should ever be used to treat patients with chronic pain, even in patients with acute pain, or patients with *subacute* pain, which if left untreated or under-treated could potentially increase the likelihood of the patient to develop chronic pain. There were often differing opinions about whether and how opioids should be used and dosed at an institutional level, at a clinic level, and in many cases even at a practice level. Additionally, there often was lack of clinical consensus at these levels about how patients should best be monitored when treated with opioid therapy, and which (if any) complementary and alternative medical treatments (e.g., cannabinoids, acupuncture, etc.) might be of potential value. In many situations, it depended on what information someone with decision-making capacity was exposed to, if they were exposed to any information at all, or mandates that forced clinicians to adhere to clinic or institutional policies about opioid prescribing. It was not uncommon for patients to be confused by a lack of consistency across practice settings because they were often essentially unaware of the pressures and logic that were impacting clinical decision-making from the regulatory, insitutional, or practice guideline perspective.

Subsequently, as the correlation between increased opioid prescribing practices and drug-related overdose fatalities grew more apparent, in addition to the flurry of guidelines targeting clinicians, there were several other "actions" which provoked reactions to "change the direction of the opioid pendulum" that followed. Many refer to these as **"silver-bullet" approaches** to reign in the relationship between opioid prescribing and the overdose epidemic gripping the United States.

One prominent silver-bullet approach was initially federal encouragement which led ultimately to mandating that states develop and maintain their own **Prescription Drug Monitoring Program (PDMP) databases**. These databases would capture information about controlled substance prescriptions to patients with one intention to be to identify people who were seeking prescriptions from multiple healthcare providers simultaneously (sometimes referred to as "drug-seeking" or "doctor shopping"). If the PDMPs were utilized regularly, the thinking was that nefarious individuals could be flagged and denied prescriptions for opioids, leading to less unintended overdoses and fatalities. In the early days, clinicians were often frustrated by the cumbersome nature of accessing these database programs, and the fact that in many cases, state PDMPs did not share data with each other, which made it difficult or impossible to identify people who straddled neighboring state lines to obtain multiple prescriptions. This has become less of an issue today, with more states sharing data with each other, but not nationally, and in many cases, just regionally. Additionally, there has been a lack of consistency with respect to the individual states requiring that the databases be checked every time a prescription for a controlled medication like an opioid is written; some states require it, others do not. Some states require that the prescriber be the person tasked with checking the PDMP, while others allow for someone else to be designated to perform this task. It is still unclear as to what the penalties are in many states for clinicians failing to comply with the PDMP requirements in those states where they exist. There has been much written in the scientific literature debating whether PDMPs have been successful in opioid risk mitigation or not, but there is little debate about the fact that by themselves, they have not been successful in being a single, "silver-bullet" solution with respect to opioid prescribing and opioid-related overdose deaths. In some cases, they have negatively impacted some clinicians' desire to prescribe opioids entirely, because not only do they capture data about patients, but they also capture data about prescribing patterns of individual clinicians. This provokes concern among prescribers about being profiled by the state medical board and/or the Drug Enforcement Administration (DEA) with respect to opioid and other controlled substance prescribing behaviors—once again creating in many cases a **fear of regulatory scrutiny**.

Many other "silver-bullet" approaches have been employed to attempt to reduce the risk of unintentional overdose related to prescribed opioids. One example was some states implementing and requiring the use of **electronic prescription systems** for controlled substance prescribing, which in some cases presented a significant barrier to clinicians who might prescribe opioid analgesics (or other controlled substances), even if the intention was to mitigate falsified or counterfeit prescriptions. Another example includes **efforts by the Drug Enforcement Administration (DEA) to limit the quantities of opioids manufactured** each year, with the presumed intention of having fewer quantities available to be prescribed to patients. Another example was the incorporation of **recommended "ceiling doses" for nonexpert clinicians treating chronic pain with opioid therapy by the Center for Disease Control and Prevention (CDC)** in their 2016 opioid prescribing guidelines [3].

Regardless of the specific actions, tactics, or strategies which were employed, the abovementioned actions, mainstream media coverage, and passionate debates regarding the overuse of opioid analgesics as a component of a pain treatment regimen were consistent in that they intended to lead to decreased opioid prescribing, or at a minimum, a higher level of discretion and/or deliberation regarding "appropriate" opioid use and likely contributed significantly to pushing "the opioid pendulum" toward "opiophobia" or a fear of prescribing.

Movement of the Pendulum and State of Paralysis in Pain Care

There are several vocal concerns which have arisen since 2020 regarding the feeling that "the opioid pendulum has swung too far." People with pain have expressed frustration over clinicians, clinics, or institutions who have either stopped prescribing opioids entirely, or strongly limited or discouraged their use, ultimately severely impacting the ability to have their opioid prescriptions renewed, refilled, or prescribed. In some cases, it has become more common even for patients on stable opioid therapy without any evidence of "red flag" behaviors or other concerns to have their opioids forcibly tapered, for exit strategies of opioid therapy to be unilaterally implemented by their prescriber, or to be told that opioids would no longer be prescribed by the practitioner moving forward. Much has been published about the reluctance of primary care clinicians to prescribe opioid analgesics to patients who they are unfamiliar with, presenting to the clinician solely for the purpose of obtaining an opioid prescription [4–6]. Additionally, publications are increasingly appearing in the literature regarding decreased opioid prescribing for patients with chronic pain related to medical conditions such as cancer, sickle-cell disease, or patients near the end of life, who would have previously been considered to be good candidates for opioid analgesic therapy.

Many clinicians who would have routinely been called upon in the past to treat patients with pain who might have been previously considered to be "appropriate" candidates for opioid analgesic therapy report that since regulators identified a relationship between the overdose epidemic and "liberal prescribing" of opioids, they have decided to step back from prescribing opioids either altogether, or to utilize them only in the most limited circumstances. In many cases, their rationale is to protect themselves from liability and regulatory scrutiny. Concerns about the "chilling effect" of regulatory efforts on opioid prescribing date back to as early as 2005 [7].

In a sense, there was and continues to be a "**state of paralysis**" which has impacted how pain is treated, how patients with pain are treated, and how opioid prescribing is perceived altogether. Things are in some ways frozen in the distant past with respect to the treatment of all but the most acute types of pain with identifiable associated pathology, with an increased sense of bias and stigma directed toward people on chronic opioid therapy, or clinicians who prescribe chronic opioid therapy. It became commonplace for patients with chronic pain being treated with opioids to feel as if they have been labeled with a "scarlet letter [8]."

An illustrative example of this paralysis involves Oxycontin® and the FDA. When Oxycontin® was reformulated in 2011 to an abuse deterrent formulation, one of the conditions of its approval by the FDA was that the manufacturer (Purdue Pharma) needed to perform clinical research to determine the efficacy of the abuse deterrent formulation in helping to mitigate the "opioid crisis" facing the United States, given Oxycontin's prominent role in contributing to the crisis. Essentially, the mandate by the FDA was to investigate and provide data to the FDA to document that changing the drug formulation to an abuse-deterrent formulation had a positive impact on the overdose epidemic. It took five years for the manufacturer and the FDA to come to agreement on the study design and protocol, and then another five years to perform the clinical trial, analyze the data, and present the findings to the FDA and its advisory committees, the Anesthetic and Analgesic Drug Products Advisory Committee to the FDA and the Drug Safety and Risk Management Advisory Committee. The manufacturer presented its findings, which seemed to indicate positive impact, but the overall sense of these advisory panels was that over the 10 years that had passed, so many other variables had impacted the crisis (such as increased availability of naloxone, the increased prevalence of fentanyl-related overdoses, etc.), that it was virtually impossible to analyze the overall positive impact on the crisis, because it did not occur "in a vacuum." This is just one example of how "paralyzed" the environment has become from a regulatory perspective, the patient's perspective, the pharmaceutical industry perspective, and from a clinical perspective.

A number of actions have been taken to try to counteract this "paralysis." One action involved the "x-waiver" DEA requirement for prescribing buprenorphine, which had been part of its Risk Evaluation and Mitigation Strategy (REMS). The x-waiver education requirement removed by President Biden in December 2022, In 2023, the FDA made the decision to make two formulations of naloxone nasal spray available over-the-counter without a prescription, and the FDA held an advisory committee meeting to evaluate a possible study protocol for a clinical trial to determine the efficacy (or lack of efficacy) of long-term opioid analgesic therapy some 10 years after making the decision to perform this kind of study. Additionally, as of June of 2023, *all clinicians* except veterinary clinicians registered with the DEA are required to participate in 8 hours of continuing education related to pain and substance use disorder assessment and treatment. Most clinicians still have little or no idea that this will be required when their DEA registration comes up for renewal. This educational requirement is a one-time requirement, implying that the DEA assumes that this mandatory activity will have a significant impact on safe prescribing, substance use treatment, and the overdose epidemic. The specific topics for this DEA-required education are relatively unclear, varied, and detailed information about acceptable education is either inconsistent, sparse, or nonexistent. At least this effort will provide some education for the many future clinicians in the course of their training who irrespective of their disciplines may receive little to none. Our training institutions do not seem to be there yet in terms of mandatory undergraduate education on these topics. There has not yet been research performed to determine if making naloxone available over the counter is scientifically resulting in preventing overdose deaths, but the sense is that it might help and the benefits outweigh the risks. There is a similar lack of evidence to support the removal of the x-waiver for buprenorphine on overdose deaths, but the sense is that it might help make buprenorphine more accessible to those in need of substance use treatment. There is also no evidence yet to show that 8 hours of a one-time educational initiative about pain and substance use disorders is a sufficient amount of education, but the sentiment seems to be that some mandated education is better than none. Reactively, a pattern of "paralysis" seems to continue, with pain patients in need increasingly frustrated about difficulties in obtaining opioid prescriptions, clinicians taking steps away from prescribing opioids, and more people dying of drug-related overdoses than ever before.

The Static Pendulum

What might be missing from the rationale of all the abovementioned actions and reactions are ways to implement clinically reproducible approaches and methodologies which do not lose sight of the need for individuality in pain assessment and pain care. Essentially, the point is that the "missing piece" might actually be the incorporation of core **ethical principles** as the basis for pain assessment, treatment plan formulation, *and* regulatory decision-making. No matter what other dynamic factors exist at the time, there is no "swinging pendulum" with respect to the role of the delivery ethically-based pain care—the use of ethics to guide pain care is a **"static pendulum."**

This does not imply that there are not challenges to the application of ethical principles to the treatment of pain. If we consider that invariably pharmacologic treatment is a de facto component of pain treatment, then safety, efficacy, and aberrant drug-related behaviors, such as nonmedical use, addiction, and diversion, must also factor into the ethical analysis. Additionally, not only does the patient as an individual need to be considered, but the other aspects of the person-with-pain's life need to be identified and considered as well. There also needs to be consideration of the fact that what is happening in the clinician's life and clinical environment can be factors which need to be considered as well, such as liability, concerns about regulatory scrutiny, institutional pressures, and anything else which could potentially impact clinical decision-making.

As mentioned previously, even though it is not actually mentioned in the Hippocratic Oath, most consider the first "rule" of medical ethics to be "**Do No Harm.**" This makes sense, especially in the context of treating people with pain. Additionally, because of the relationship between opioid analgesics, addiction, and the overdose epidemic, the desire to "do no harm" must also apply to potential harm to people *other than* the patient; it must apply to other members of the household, members of community, and to members of society.

Drivers of ethical decision-making in pain management can be conscious, subconscious, or both. They will often include limitation of knowledge (e.g., lack of education), because clinicians typically recommend courses of treatment that they are familiar with, based upon previous clinical experiences, cognitive and precognitive biases, and the four core ethical principles: **autonomy, justice, nonmaleficence, and beneficence.** This may seem a bit simplistic, and easy to follow, but sometimes that may not be the case. Determining which ethical principle(s) should take priority in guiding clinician decision-making can sometimes be challenging, especially when prescription pain medications such as opioid analgesics are considered as part of the pain treatment plan. There may be situations where the core principles themselves overlap given the individual circumstances, and there may also be times when they conflict with each other. While it might be desirable to have, there should be an simple algorithm for weighing and balancing these conflicts, sometimes significantly more effort is required—**but it *is* worth the effort.**

To deliver ethical pain care irrespective of the dynamic nature of the clinical, social, or regulatory environment, pain care must place emphasis on respect for the patient, preserving their dignity, considering their emotional state, incorporating mutually-determined realistic goals and expectations, and maintaining privacy, confidentiality, and, above all, integrity. Communication is a key ingredient to ethical decision-making and must go beyond the cursory history and physical. Inquiry needs to be made about needs, desires, social determinants, and other factors which may inform not only life context, but potential risk(s), not only at the patient level, but also within the patient's social circle and community setting. **Motivational interviewing** can assist with determining relevant and potential aspects of the patient context to ensure safety and efficacy. Identifying a pathophysiologic basis for pain is ideal, but sometimes not achievable. That does not mean that **establishing a diagnosis or at a minimum differential diagnosis** is not as critical to the delivery of ethical pain care as setting **realistic goals and expectations that are individualized and collaborative** in nature.

Ethically judicious consideration of opioid analgesics does not mean avoiding prescribing them; it means thoughtfully and rationally considering them, making sure that responsibilities are clearly communicated and understood by all parties involved. There should always be an ethical analysis of the indications related to prescribing an opioid and mitigating potential harm(s) related to their use. This ethical analysis and rationale should routinely be documented in the patient's medical record. This requires willingness on the part of clinicians, their clinical settings, regulators, and other stakeholders to make the ethical analysis a core part of the pain assessment and treatment process. A mandate to deliver ethical pain care with the goal of achieving the best possible outcomes along with the mission of delivering that care with safety, fairness, equity, compassion, empathy, and minimization of potential harm(s) is a pendulum that will never swing.

References

1. Gourlay DL, Heit HA, Almahrezi A. Universal precautions in pain medicine: a rational approach to the treatment of chronic pain. Pain Med. 2005;6(2):107–12.
2. Chou R, Fanciullo GJ, Fine PG, Adler JA, Ballantyne JC, Davies P, Donovan MI, Fishbain DA, Foley KM, Fudin J, Gilson AM, Kelter A, Mauskop A, O'Connor PG, Passik SD, Pasternak GW, Portenoy RK, Rich BA, Roberts RG, Todd KH, Miaskowski C. American Pain Society-American Academy of Pain Medicine Opioids Guidelines Panel. Clinical guidelines for the use of chronic opioid therapy in chronic noncancer pain. J Pain. 2009;10(2):113–30.
3. Dowell D, Haegerich TM, Chou R. CDC guideline for prescribing opioids for chronic pain – United States, 2016. MMWR Recomm Rep. 2016;65(1):1–49.
4. Danielson EC, Harle CA, Downs SM, Militello L, Mazurenko O. How opioid prescribing policies influence primary care clinicians' treatment decisions and conversations with patients with chronic pain. J Opioid Manag. 2021;17(6):499–509.
5. Tong ST, Hochheimer CJ, Brooks EM, Sabo RT, Jiang V, Day T, Rozman JS, Kashiri PL, Krist AH. Chronic opioid prescribing in primary care: factors and perspectives. Ann Fam Med. 2019;17(3):200–6.
6. Knight KR, Kushel M, Chang JS, Zamora K, Ceasar R, Hurstak E, Miaskowski C. Opioid pharmacovigilance: a clinical-social history of the changes in opioid prescribing for patients with co-occurring chronic non-cancer pain and substance use. Soc Sci Med. 2017;186:87–95.
7. Schmidt C. Experts worry about chilling effect of federal regulations on treating pain. JNCI J Natl Cancer Inst. 2005;97(8):554–5. https://doi.org/10.1093/jnci/97.8.554. Accessed 31 July 2023.
8. Benintendi A, Kosakowski S, Lagisetty P, Larochelle M, Bohnert ASB, Bazzi AR. "I felt like I had a scarlet letter": recurring experiences of structural stigma surrounding opioid tapers among patients with chronic, non-cancer pain. Drug Alcohol Depend. 2021;1(222):108664.

Index

© The Editor(s) (if applicable) and The Author(s), under exclusive license to Springer
Nature Switzerland AG 2024
K. L. Zacharoff, P. Migdal, *Pain, Drugs, and Ethics*,
https://doi.org/10.1007/978-3-031-63018-7

Printed by Printforce, the Netherlands